INTERFERON ALPHA-2: PRE-CLINICAL AND CLINICAL EVALUATION

DEVELOPMENTS IN ONCOLOGY

F.J. Cleton and J.W.I.M. Simons, eds., Genetic Origins of Tumour Cells.
ISBN 90-247-2272-1
J. Aisner and P. Chang, eds., Cancer Treatment Research. ISBN 90-247-2358-2
B.W. Ongerboer de Visser, D.A. Bosch and W.M.H. van Woerkom-Eykenboom, eds.,
Neuro-oncology: Clinical and Experimental Aspects. ISBN 90-247-2421-X
K. Hellmann, P. Hilgard and S. Eccles, eds., Metastasis: Clinical and Experimental Aspects. ISBN 90-247-2424-4
H.F. Seigler, ed., Clinical Management of Melanoma. ISBN 90-247-2584-4
P. Correa and W. Haenszel, eds., Epidemiology of Cancer of the Digestive Tract.
ISBN 90-247-2601-8
L.A. Liotta and I.R. Hart, eds., Tumour Invasion and Metastasis. ISBN 90-247-2611-5
J. Bánóczy, ed., Oral Leukoplakia. ISBN 90-247-2655-7
C. Tijssen, M. Halprin and L. Endtz, eds., Familial Brain Tumours. ISBN 90-247-2691-3
F.M. Muggia, C.W. Young and S.K. Carter, eds., Anthracycline Antibiotics in Cancer.
ISBN 90-247-2711-1
B.W. Hancock, ed., Assessment of Tumour Response. ISBN 90-247-2712-X
D.E. Peterson, ed., Oral Complications of Cancer Chemotherapy. ISBN 0-89838-563-6
R. Mastrangelo, D.G. Poplack and R. Riccardi, eds., Central Nervous System Leukemia.
Prevention and Treatment. ISBN 0-89838-570-9
A. Polliack, ed., Human Leukemias. Cytochemical and Ultrastructural Techniques in
Diagnosis and Research. ISBN 0-89838-585-7
W. Davis, C. Maltoni and S. Tanneberger, eds., The Control of Tumor Growth and its
Biological Bases. ISBN 0-89838-603-9
A.P.M. Heintz, C.Th. Griffiths and J.B. Trimbos, eds., Surgery in Gynecological Oncology. ISBN 0-89838-604-7
M.P. Hacker, E.B. Double and I. Krakoff, eds., Platinum Coordination Complexes in
Cancer Chemotherapy. ISBN 0-89838-619-5
M.J. van Zwieten, The Rat as Animal Model in Breast Cancer Research: A Histopathological Study of Radiation- and Hormone-Induced Rat Mammary Tumors.
ISBN 0-89838-624-1
B. Löwenberg and A. Hagenbeek, eds., Minimal Residual Disease in Acute Leukemia.
ISBN 0-89838-630-6
I. van der Waal and G.B. Snow, eds., Oral Oncology. ISBN 0-89838-631-4
B.W. Hancock and A.H. Ward, eds., Immunological Aspects of Cancer.
ISBN 0-89838-664-0
K.V. Honn and B.F. Sloane, Hemostatic Mechanisms and Metastasis. ISBN 0-89838-667-5
K.R. Harrap, W. Davis and A.H. Calvert, eds., Cancer Chemotherapy and Selective Drug
Development. ISBN 0-89838-673-X
C.J.H. van de Velde and P.H. Sugarbaker, eds., Liver Metastasis. ISBN 0-89838-648-5
D.J. Ruiter, K. Welvaart and S. Ferrone, eds., Cutaneous Melanoma and Precursor Lesions. ISBN 0-89838-689-6
S.B. Howell, ed., Intra-arterial and Intracavitary Cancer Chemotherapy.
ISBN 0-89838-691-8
D.L. Kisner and J.F. Smyth, eds., Interferon Alpha-2: Pre-Clinical and Clinical Evaluation. ISBN 0-89838-701-9

INTERFERON ALPHA-2: PRE-CLINICAL AND CLINICAL EVALUATION

Proceedings of the Symposium held in Adjunction with the Second International Conference on Malignant Lymphoma, Lugano, Switzerland, June 13, 1984

edited by

Daniel L. KISNER
Dept. of Medicine, Div. of Oncology
University of Texas
Health Science Center at San Antonio
San Antonio, Texas
USA

J.F. SMYTH
Dept. of Clinical Oncology
University of Edinburgh
Western General Hospital
Edinburgh
Scotland

1985 **MARTINUS NIJHOFF PUBLISHERS**
a member of the KLUWER ACADEMIC PUBLISHERS GROUP
BOSTON / DORDRECHT / LANCASTER

Distributors

for the United States and Canada: Kluwer Academic Publishers, 190 Old Derby Street, Hingham, MA 02043, USA
for the UK and Ireland: Kluwer Academic Publishers, MTP Press Limited, Falcon House, Queen Square, Lancaster LA1 1RN, UK
for all other countries: Kluwer Academic Publishers Group, Distribution Center, P.O. Box 322, 3300 AH Dordrecht, The Netherlands

Library of Congress Cataloging in Publication Data

```
Interferon alpha-2

  (Developments in oncology)
  1. Cancer--Chemotherapy--Evaluation--Congresses.
2. Interferon--Therapeutic use--Congresses. 3. Drugs--
Testing--Congresses. I. Kisner, D. II. Smyth, John F.
III. International Conference on Malignant Lymphoma
(2nd : 1984 : Lugano, Switzerland) IV. Title: Interferon
alpha-two. V. Series. (DNLM: 1. Drug Evaluation--
congresses. 2. Drug screening--congresses. 3. Interferon
Type I--congresses. W1 DE998N / QV 268.5 I607 1984)

RC271.I46I55  1985   616.99'4061   84-27166
ISBN 0-89838-701-9
```

ISBN 0-89838-701-9 (this volume)

Copyright

PRINTED IN THE NETHERLANDS

Table of Contents

Preface

List of Contributors

Preface

Interferon alpha-2 is a genetically engineered, highly purified pharmaceutical agent that has undergone extensive phase I and phase II clinical study in more than 1000 patients. The material has biological activity by intravenous, intramuscular and subcutaneous routes. Clinical toxicity principally involves the 'influenza like' syndrome previously seen with native interferons. Other important toxicities include anorexia, hepatitis, confusion and myelosuppression. Tolerable doses in multiple schedules and routes of administration have been determined.

Phase II clinical trials with multiple routes and schedules of administration have been performed. Significant clinical activity has been found in non-Hodgkin's lymphomas (both low grade and high grade), refractory and relapsing multiple myeloma, hairy cell leukemia, Kaposi's sarcoma, with suggestions of activity in Hodgkin's disease, renal cell carcinoma, and melanoma.

The studies performed to date have for the most part involved small numbers of heavily pre-treated patients. Large-scale clinical trials in some of these diseases are now warranted in populations of patients with as little bulk disease and prior treatment as is feasible for each tumour type. This is particularly the case in Hodgkin's disease and subcategories of the non-Hodgkin's lymphomas. Alternately, interferon alpha-2 might be used to maintain remissions induced by other modalities (i.e., in NHL, multiple myeloma, ovarian cancer). In some advanced disease settings, combinations of interferon alpha-2 with chemotherapeutic agents should now be investigated. Studies with the human tumour cloning assay and the nude mouse xenograft system suggest that interferon alpha-2 might be synergistic with doxorubicin, cis-platinum and vinblastine. One clinical trial combining doxorubicin with interferon alpha-2 has been initiated with good tolerance, and antitumour activity demonstrated in cervical cancer, ovarian cancer, and pancreatic cancer.

More phase I combination protocols are required, using doxorubicin, vinblastine and cis-platinum prior to broad phase II testing. Phase III randomised comparisons will be required to clearly define the comparative efficacy of the interferon alpha-2 combinations. Tumour types of interest for such combinations include multiple myeloma, non-Hodgkin's lymphomas, Hodgkin's disease, Kaposi's sarcoma, and possibly cervical and ovarian cancer.

If tumour burden is relevant to the effect of interferon alpha-2 as seems possible, one additional area where interferon alpha-2 should be studied is the surgical adjuvant situation where a minimal tumour burden is present. Despite only modest response data, renal cell carcinoma and melanoma are reasonable tumours for such trials.

Work to characterise the cell surface receptor for interferon alpha-2 suggests the possibility of selecting patients with the most likelihood of clinical response. Given the clinical toxicity of interferon alpha-2, such selection would spare inappropriate therapy for some patients.

Other future areas of research interest include intracavitary therapy, combinations with radiotherapy and the evaluation of other interferons. Interferon alpha-2 is still an experimental therapy, and several more years of large-scale trials will be required to clearly define its role in clinical oncology.

DANIEL KISNER, M.D., SAN ANTONIO, TEXAS

JOHN SMYTH, M.D., EDINBURGH, SCOTLAND

List of Contributors

E. BONNEM, Associate Director, Oncology Clinical Research, Schering Corporation, Kenilworth, NJ 07033, USA

M.R. COOPER, Professor of Medicine, Bowman Gray School of Medicine, 300 So. Hawthorne Road, Winston-Salem, NC 27103, USA

J.J. COSTANZI, Professor, Chief Division Hematology-Oncology, Department of Medicine, The University of Texas Medical Branch, MW414, 9th and Market Sts., Galveston, TX 77550, USA

D. CROWTHER, Professor, Cancer Research Campaign, Chair of Medical Oncology, Manchester University, Christie Hospital and Holt Radium Institute, Wilmslow Road Withington, Manchester, M20 9BX, UK

R.W. FERRARESI, Associate Medical Director, Research Division, Schering Corporation, Kenilworth, NJ 07033, USA

H.M. GOLOMB, Professor, Department of Medicine, Chief, Section of Hematology/Oncology, University of Chicago, Pritzker School of Medicine, Box 420, 950 East 59th St., Chicago, IL 60637, USA

N.C. GORIN, Professor, Hematology and Internal Medicine, C.H.U. Saint-Antoine, University of Paris VI, 184 Rue du Faubourg St. Antoine, 75012 Paris, Cedex 12, France

M. GRIMM, Medical Research Associate, Research Division, Schering Corporation, Kenilworth, NJ 07033, USA

H. HOST, Professor, Head, Department of Oncology, The Norwegian Radium Hospital, Montebello, Oslo 3, Norway

R.S. KAPLAN, Associate Professor of Medicine and Oncology, University of Maryland Cancer Center, 22 South Greene Street, Baltimore, MD 21201, USA

C. KARANES, Associate Professor of Medicine, Harper Grace Hospital, Wayne State University, 3990 John R. Blvd., Detroit, MI 48201, USA

D.L. KISNER, Associate Professor of Medicine, Dept. of Medicine, Division of Oncology, The University of Texas, Health Sciences Center at San Antonio, 7703 Floyd Curl Drive, San Antonio, TX 78284, USA

R.D. LEAVITT, Assistant Professor of Medicine and Oncology, University of Maryland Cancer Center, 22 South Greene Street, Baltimore, MD 21201, USA

P.J. LEIBOWITZ, Associate Director, Department of Molecular Biology, Schering Corporation, 60 Orange Street, Bloomfield, NJ 07003, USA

C.F. LEONARD, Honorary Consultant, Senior Lecturer, Department of Clinical Oncology, University of Edinburgh, Edinburgh, EH4 2XU, UK

T.M. MORGAN, Assistant Professor of Community Medicine, Bowman Gray School of Medicine, Wake Forest University, 300 South Hawthorne Road, Winston-Salem, NC 27103, USA

H.B. MUSS, Associate Professor of Medicine, Hematology/Oncology, Bowman Gray School of Medicine, Wake Forest University, 300 South Hawthorne Road, Winston-Salem, NC 27103, USA

T.L. NAGABHUSHAN, Director Medicinal and Protein Chemistry, Senior Research Fellow, Schering Corporation, 60 Orange Street, Bloomfield, NJ 07003, USA

H. OZER, Associate Chief, Department of Medical Oncology, Roswell Park Memorial Institute, 666 Elm Street, Buffalo, NY 14263, USA

R.B. POLLARD, Assistant Professor of Internal Medicine and Microbiology, The University of Texas Medical Branch, 5-17 McCullough Bldg., Galveston TX 77550, USA

C. PORTLOCK, Associate Professor of Medicine, Section of Medical Oncology, Yale University, 333 Cedar Street, New Haven, CT 06510, USA

M.J. RATAIN, Research Associate, Department of Medicine, Section of Hematology/Oncology, University of Chicago, Pritzker School of Medicine, Box 420, 950 East 59th Street, Chicago, IL 60637, USA

V. RATANATHARATHORN, Assistant Professor of Medicine, Division of Oncology, Harper Grace Hospital, Wayne State University, 3990 John R. Blvd., Detroit, MI 48201, USA

S. RUDNICK, Vice President Clinical Research, Biogen Research Corporation, 14 Cambridge Center, Cambridge, MA 02142, USA

J.H. SCARFFE, Honorary Consultant, Senior Lecturer, Cancer Research Campaign, Department of Medical Oncology, Manchester University, Christie Hospital and Holt Radium Institute, Wilmslow Road Withington, Manchester, M20 9BX, UK

J.F. SMYTH, Professor and ICRF Chair of Medical Oncology, University of Edinburgh, Head, Department of Clinical Oncology, Western General Hospital, Edinburgh EH4 2XU, UK

R.J. SPIEGEL, Director, Oncology Clinical Research, Schering Corporation, Kenilworth, NJ 07033, USA

P.P. TROTTA, Research Fellow Chemical Research, Schering Corporation, 60 Orange Street, Bloomfield, NJ 07003, USA

J.E. ULTMANN, Professor of Medicine, Cancer Research Center, University of Chicago, Box 444, 950 East 59th Street, Chicago, IL 60637, USA

J. WAGSTAFF, Research Fellow, Cancer Research Campaign, Department of Medical Oncology, Manchester University, Christie Hospital and Holt Radium Insitute, Wilmslow Road Withington, Manchester, M20 9BX, UK

C.E. WELANDER, Assistant Professor, Obstetrics and Gynecology, Bowman Gray School of Medicine, Wake Forest University, 300 South Hawthorne Road, Winston-Salem, NC 27103, USA

1. Recombinant DNA Technology and Characterization of Recombinant Alpha-2 Interferon

T.L. NAGABHUSHAN and P.J. LEIBOWITZ

Abstract

The strain of *E. coli,* KMAC-43, used for the large-scale production of alpha-2 interferon was engineered at Schering by Leibowitz and his co-workers. The alpha-2 interferon gene used in this construction was obtained from a cDNA clone, Hif-SN206, developed by Weissmann. The large-scale method developed in our laboratory for the purification of alpha-2 interferon from the bacterial extracts produces highly pure, crystalline alpha-2 interferon which is dissolved in 20 mM phosphate buffer at neutral pH to constitute bulk drug solution that is used in various formulations.

The protein has been thoroughly characterized using physico-chemical and biological methods. The average specific activity of clinical grade alpha-2 interferon is 1.7×10^8 u/mgP. The purity of the product has been established by reversed phase HPLC (>98% pure), amino acid analysis, amino acid sequencing, circular dichroism spectrometry, ultracentrifugation, SDS-PAGE and 2-D gel electrophoresis. Details of these methods and results will be discussed.

Introduction

In this article we review the collaborative works of several scientists from Schering Corporation, U.S.A. and Dr. Charles Weissmann's laboratory in Switzerland. The construction of a typical plasmid for the expression of human recombinant alpha-2 interferon in *E. coli* as well as the physico-chemical and biological properties of the protein are discussed.

Alpha-2 interferon producing strains

The strain of *E. coli* used for the production of recombinant human alpha-2 interferon for world-wide clinical trials was engineered at Schering Corporation, U.S.A. and contains the plasmid KMAC-43. The interferon gene in KMAC-43 was originally obtained from derivatives of an earlier construction, Hif-SN 206, of Weissmann and coworkers [1, 2]. The vector in Hif-SN 206 is pBR322. The IFN coding sequence of Hif-SN 206 is preceded by 51 nucleotides that are part of a signal sequence preceding the mature coding sequence in the human genome [2, 3]. Weissmann and his coworkers removed the remnant of the signal sequence of this interferon alpha-2 cDNA by fusing a lac promoter to the first codon of the mature coding sequence using a cloning strategy in which the sequence coding for the mature protein would be preceded by a translation initiation codon. This plasmid is designated AUG/206-1.

A brief summary of the construction of AUG/206-1 is depicted diagrammatically in Fig. 1. The 203 base pair Hae III fragment of the lac operon was digested with Alu 1 to obtain the regulatory region. This was ligated to a custom-made Eco RI linker fragment containing a translational start signal. After digestion with Eco RI and S_1, a promoter-operator fragment was generated that contained an initiator codon at its carboxy terminal end. The coding sequence of alpha-2 interferon cDNA was cleaved at the Sau 3a site located between the codon for the first and second amino acid of the mature interferon sequence, and the Hind III linker was ligated to the cleaved end, reconstructing the first codon and adding a Hind III cleavage site. The two ends, i.e. the promoter-operator fragment and the fragment containing the mature alpha-2 coding sequence were joined with DNA ligase to yield a sequence encoding mature interferon preceded by a methionine. The strain of *E. coli* containing the above plasmid, AUG/206-1, produced about 1 mg of alpha-2 interferon per liter of culture [4]. About 50 percent of the interferon molecules lost the methionine residue by post-translational cleavage [4].

In order to improve the yield of alpha-2 interferon, Weissmann and coworkers [4] constructed another strain, MISH-21b, with the alpha-2 interferon gene fused to the β-lactamase promoter of the pBR322 vector. The fusion was done in such a manner that the first ATG triplet was followed directly by the first codon of mature interferon (cysteine).

The yield of alpha-2 interferon in the MISH-21b fermentation was greatly improved over that of Aug/206-1 [4]. It was also found that greater than 90% of the interferon molecules did not contain N-terminal methionine [5] and that all of the intracellular interferon is soluble. KMAC-43 is a vastly superior producer, providing intra-cellularly soluble interferon without statistically meaningful levels of N-terminal methionine.

Physico-chemical characterization of human recombinant alpha-2 interferon

The large-scale method for the selective extraction of alpha-2 interferon from the cells and its purification was developed at Schering Corporation U.S.A.

Figure 3 shows crystals of alpha-2 interferon obtained from a typical purification scheme. The shape and size of the crystals vary depending upon the conditions of crystallization [7].

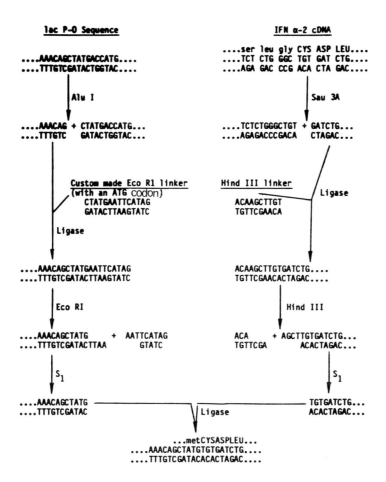

Figure 1. Summary construction of AUG/206-1.

The purity of interferon by HPLC analysis is shown in Fig. 4. The analysis was performed using a Waters Associates u-Bondapak C-18 column (30 cm x 3.9 mm) and a gradient of 31.4% to 62.7% aqueous acetonitrile (90%) containing O.01M TFA at 1 ml/min, over 30 min [8]. The protein was detected by fluorescent monitoring after post-column derivatization with ortho-phthalaldehyde [9].

Table 1 shows typical results for amino acid analysis of alpha-2 interferon and in this particular case we have taken the average of 15 batches. As seen, the agreement between experimental and theoretical values on a mole percent basis is excellent. The method used for determining the amino acid composition involved acid hydrolysis of the protein with 6.7N hydrochloric acid *in vacuo* for 18 h at 160°C followed by chromatographic analysis of the digest on an ES Industries C-18 column (15 cm × 4.6 mm) utilizing paired ion chromatography as modified by Hatch and Radjai [10]. The amino acids were detected by fluorescent monitoring of ortho-phthalaldehyde post-column derivatives. Cysteine (cys-

4

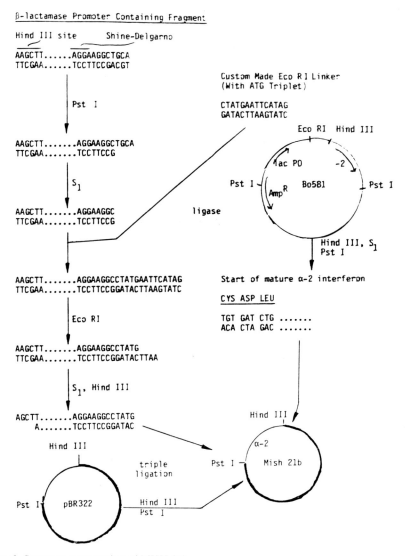

Figure 2. Summary construction of MISH 21b.

tine) and tryptophan were not quantitated due to their destruction during the hydrolysis. Proline was not detected since it does not form a fluorescent derivative with ortho-phthalaldehyde.

We have used two techniques for obtaining the amino acid sequence of the alpha-2 interferon protein. In the first, using a gas phase sequencer, Model 470A, Applied Biosystems Inc., sequencing was performed from the N-terminal through 57 amino acid residues [11]. The protein was subjected to reduction with dithiothreitol and alkylated with iodoacetamide to allow subsequent indentification of cysteine residues [12]. Sequencing was also performed without reducing

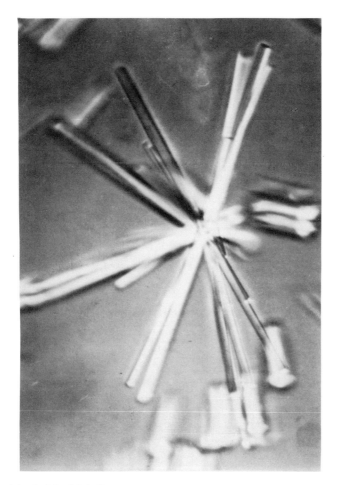

Figure 3. Crystals of alpha-2 interferon.

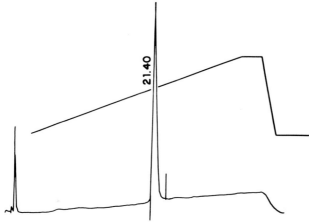

Figure 4. HPLC of alpha-2 interferon.

Table 1. Amino acid composition of alpha-2 interferon.

Amino acid	Theoretical mole percent	Average mole percent
Asx	7.74	9.06 ± 0.46
Ser	9.03	10.33 ± 0.48
Gly	3.23	3.80 ± 0.91
Glx	16.77	19.03 ± 0.79
Thr	6.45	5.54 ± 0.58
Ala	5.16	5.61 ± 0.58
Val	4.52	2.62 ± 0.23
Met	3.23	2.82 ± 0.59
Tyr	3.23	2.81 ± 0.45
Ile	5.16	3.52 ± 0.39
Leu	13.55	13.96 ± 0.46
Phe	6.45	6.51 ± 0.20
His	1.94	1.95 ± 0.15
Lys	7.10	6.53 ± 0.58
Arg	6.45	5.99 ± 0.70

the disulfide bonds and alkylating the protein. The phenylthiohydantoin amino acids were analyzed by HPLC on an IBM cyanopropyl silane column using 0.02 M sodium acetate, pH 6.2 with an organic eluting solvent, acetonitrile: methanol 4:1. The first 57 amino acids are in agreement with those predicted from the cDNA nucleotide sequence [2] (see Fig. 5).

Similar sequencing of fragments of alpha-2 interferon obtained after cleavage with cyanogen bromide [13] and isolation of the pure fragments by HPLC also confirmed the sequence.

Thus, we have determined the sequence of the protein for amino acids 1 through 57, 60 through 86, 88 through 97, 99–100, 102–103, 113 through 137, 139 through 146 and 149 through 164. Since the last amino acid (glu) could not be detected by the Edman degradation method, we performed tryptic digestion of the C-terminal cyanogen bromide fragment. Based on amino acid sequence and enzyme specificity [14], this treatment is expected to yield a peptide of 13 amino acids, a tripeptide (ser-lys-glu) and a free amino acid, arginine. The digest was fractionated by HPLC and the fraction containing the tripeptide and arginine was subjected to amino acid analysis. The only four amino acids detected were ser, lys, glu and arg which confirms the presence of glu in the terminal tripeptide.

In the second technique, which is still in a developmental stage we employed gas chromatography/mass spectrometry (GC/MS) sequence survey of alpha-2 interferon after subjecting the protein to non-specific cleavage with subtilisin followed by trifluoroacetylation and permethylation [15]. This experiment was done at the University of Geneva in Professor Robin Offord's laboratory under the supervision of Drs. Offord and Keith Rose. The sample was dissolved in

CYS	ASP	LEU	PRO	GLN	THR	HIS	SER	LEU	GLY	SER	ARG	ARG	THR	LEU
MET	LEU	LEU	ALA	GLN	MET	ARG	ARG	ILE	SER	LEU	PHE	SER	CYS	LEU
LYS	ASP	ARG	HIS	ASP	PHE	GLY	PHE	PRO	GLN	GLU	GLU	PHE	GLY	ASN
GLN	PHE	GLN	LYS	ALA	GLU	THR	ILE	PRO	VAL	LEU	HIS	GLU	MET	ILE
GLN	GLN	ILE	PHE	ASN	LEU	PHE	SER	THR	LYS	ASP	SER	SER	ALA	ALA
TRP	ASP	GLU	THR	LEU	LEU	ASP	LYS	PHE	TYR	THR	GLU	LEU	TYR	GLN
GLN	LEU	ASN	ASP	LEU	GLU	ALA	CYS	VAL	ILE	GLN	GLY	VAL	GLY	VAL
THR	GLU	THR	PRO	LEU	MET	LYS	GLU	ASP	SER	ILE	LEU	ALA	VAL	ARG
LYS	TYR	PHE	GLN	ARG	ILE	THR	LEU	TYR	LEU	LYS	GLU	LYS	LYS	TYR
SER	PRO	CYS	ALA	TRP	GLU	VAL	VAL	ARG	ALA	GLU	ILE	MET	ARG	SER
PHE	SER	LEU	SER	THR	ASN	LEU	GLN	GLU	SER	LEU	ARG	SER	LYS	GLU

Figure 5. Sequence of alpha-2 interferon.
(———— EDMAN ------ GC/MS)

deionized 8M urea containing 0.5M ammonium carbonate and 4% W/V SDS. The solution was dialyzed against water at 4°C and then lyophilized. 0.2 mg of the lyophilized powder was taken up in 50 μl subtilisin for 4 h at 37°C. The digest was lyophilized, then derivatized by trifluoroacetylation and permethylation. Approximately 1/5th of the product was used for GC/MS analysis. The peptides identified by this technique are shown in Fig. 5 which includes a similar survey of the C-terminal cyanogen bromide fragment.

The average apparent molecular weight of alpha-2 interferon was found to be 18,500 $\pm$ 600 from one-dimensional SDS-PAGE [16] (Fig. 6). The $\pm$ 600 standard deviation is a gel to gel variation. The apparent molecular weight obtained is in good agreement with 19,271 calculated from the amino acid sequence. The homogeneity of the protein is apparent from the single band seen even after staining with silver [17].

As seen in Fig. 7, there is excellent correlation between the location of bioactivity and the mobility of the major species on SDS-PAGE. In this case SDS-PAGE was conducted under non-reducing conditions.

The two-dimensional gel electrophoresis of alpha-2 interferon showed one major band and this is shown in Fig. 8 [18].

Circular dichroism (CD) spectra of alpha-2 interferon as obtained on a Jasco J-500A CD Spectropolarimeter with a DP-500N data processor are shown in Fig. 9. The spectra were run on samples diluted in 20 mM phosphate buffer at pH. 7 to yield a final concentration of 0.16 mg/ml, as determined by Lowry assay. The near and far UV spectra are corrected for baseline variation and are normalized

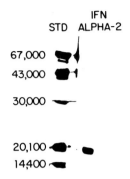

Figure 6. SDS-PAGE of alpha-2 interferon.

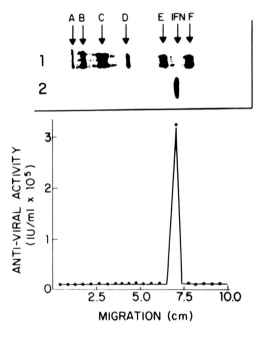

Figure 7. Correlation of biological activity of alpha-2 interferon with gel mobility.

to $^{\theta}0.01\%$. The values for $^{\theta}0.01\%$ at five significant wavelengths are:

(nm)	1 cm	Chromophore
291	−1.22	Tryptophan
286	−1.16	Tryptophan
233	−14.3	Unknown
218	−139.0	α-helix
208	−144.0	α-helix

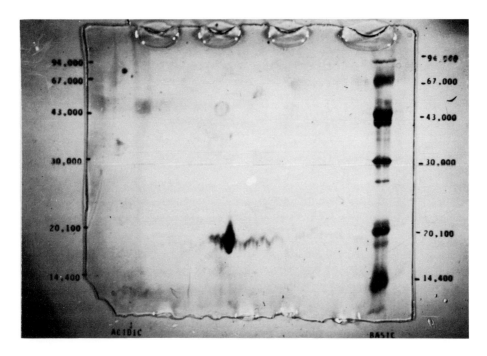

Figure 8. Two-dimensional gel of alpha-2 interferon.

The negative bands in the near UV at 291 and 286 nm are due to the highly asymmetric tryptophan chromophore. The 233 nm shoulder is characteristic of alpha-2 interferon; the nature of the chromophores that contribute to this dichroism is unknown.

The far UV data at 208 and 218 nm were evaluated using the methods of Chen [19, 20] and Greenfield [21] for computing protein conformation from CD spectra. The conformation parameters obtained are consistent with those predicted from the amino acid sequence using the Chou and Fasman rules [22-24]. Our results are very similar to the ones published by Bewley, Levine and Wetzel [25] for Genetech's cloned alpha interferon.

Fig. 10 shows the sedimentation velocity profile of alpha-2 interferon measured in the ultraviolet at 280 nm under two different solvent conditons. The experiments were performed at Cornell Medical Center using a Beckman Model E analytical ultracentrifuge. Alpha-2 interferon forms an aggregate in solution at a concentration of 0.7 mg/ml in phosphate buffer at neutral pH, as implied by its sedimentation coefficient of 4.82S (panel A). The aggregates are readily dissociated when the ionic strength of the medium is increased; for example, the sedimentation coefficient drops to 1.95S when 1.0 sodium chloride is included in the buffer, as observed in panel B.

The specific activity of alpha-2 interferon has been determined by two means. First, the anti-viral activity was determined by a cytopathic effect (CPE) inhibi-

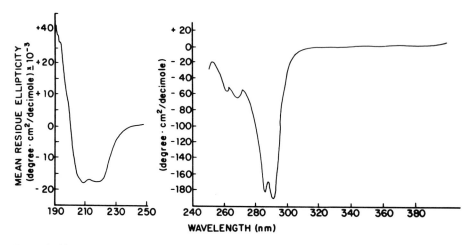

Figure 9. Circular dichroism of alpha-2 interferon.

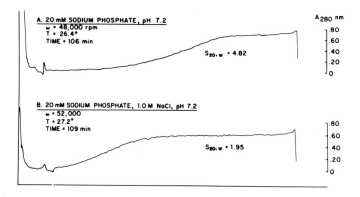

Figure 10. Sedimentation velocity of alpha-2 interferon.

tion assay using human foreskin diploid fibroblasts and EMC virus (ATCC-VR-129) and protein concentration was obtained by Lowry assay using human serum albumin as standard. Second, the specific activity was evaluated by radioimmunoassay (RIA) employing polystyrene bead immobilized polyclonal antibodies to α-interferon and iodinated monoclonal NK-2 antibodies [26]. Table 2 contains a summary of the values for specific activity calculated by CPE and RIA. The mean value for 35 batches was $(1.72 \pm 0.1) \times 10^8$ IU/mg protein by CPE and $(1.70 \pm 0.08) \times 10^8$ IU/mg protein by RIA.

Antiviral activity of recombinant human alpha-2 interferon

In Table 3 the *in vitro* antiviral activity of alpha-2 interferon against a number of viruses is given. As seen, alpha-2 interferon is most active against rhinovirus in

Table 2. Correlation of RIA-CPE-Protein Assays (17 Batches).

Test methods	Correlation coefficient
RIA-Protein	0.949
RIA-CPE	0.937
CPE-Protein	0.927

Table 3. In vitro antiviral activity of IFN alpha-2.

Challenge virus	Host cell	TCID^{50} units/ml
Rhinovirus	MRC-5*	$1.0 \times 10^1 - 6.2 \times 10^2$
Coronavirus	WI-38*	1.0×10^3
Respiratory syncytial	HEP-2**	1.0×10^3
Herpes simplex (I)	WI-38*	1.2×10^4
Vaccina	WI-38*	4.0×10^4
Herpes simplex (II)	WI-38*	3.5×10^5
Varicella-Zoster	WI-38*	5.0×10^5
Cytomegalovirus	WI-38*	3.0×10^6
Adenovirus	HEP-2**	5.0×10^7

* Lung
** Nasopharyngeal

the lung cell line. It is also very potent against coronavirus and respiratory syncytial virus. While its potency is moderate against the Herpes type viruses, it is inactive against adenovirus.

Acknowledgements

The authors wish to thank Dr. C. Weissmann and his staff (Molecular Biology), Dr. P. Trotta and his staff (Protein Chemistry), Dr. M. Finkelstein and his staff (Molecular Biology), Dr. H. Surprenant and his staff (Quality Control), Dr. J. Schwartz, Mr. E. Oden and their staff (Assays) for results presented in this manuscript.

References

1. Weissmann C, Nagata S, Boll W, Foutoulakis M, Fujisawa A, Fujisawa JI, Haynes J, Henco K, Mantei N, Ragg H, Schein C, Schmid J, Shaw G, Streuli M, Taira H, Todokoro K, Weidle U: Structure and expressions of human alpha-interferon genes. Abstr. ICN-UCLA Symposium on Chemistry and Biology of Interferons: Relationship to Therapeutics, 1982.
2. Streuli M, Nagata S, Weissmann C: Science 209:1343, 1980.
3. Nagata S, Taira H, Hall A, Johnsrud L, Streuli M, Escodi J, Boll W, Cantell K, Weissmann C: Nature 284:27, 1980.

12

4. Weissmann C: Interferon 3. Academic Press, 1981, p. 102.
5. Nagabhushan TL, Bond M: unpublished results.
6. Leibowitz P, *et al*: U.S. Patent 4, 315, 852, 1982.
7. Nagabhushan TL, Le HV, Kosecki R, Reichert P, Sharma B, Trotta P: unpublished results.
8. Bennett HPJ, Browne CA, Solomon S: Liq. Chrom 3 (9): 1353, 1980.
9. Benson JR, Hare PE: Proc. Nat Acad Sci USA 72 (2): 619 1975.
10. Hatch RT, Radjai M: J Chromatography 196:319, 1980.
11. Hunkapiller MW, Hood LE: Science 207:523, 1980.
12. Bond M: unpublished results.
13. Gross E, Witkop B: J Biol Chem 237:1856, 1962.
14. Mihalyi E: Application of Proteolytic Enzymes to Protein Structure Studies, 2nd ed., Vol. I, 1978, p. 142.
15. Rose K, Priddle JD, Offord RE, Esnouf MP: J Biochem 187: 239-243, 1980.
16. Laemmli UK: Nature 227:680, 1970.
17. Oakley BR, *et al*: Analyt Biochem, 105:361, 1980.
18. O'Farrell P: J Biol Chem 250 (10): 4007, 1975.
19. Chen YH *et al*: Biochemistry 11:4120, 1972.
20. Chen YH *et al*: Biochemistry 13:3350, 1974.
21. Greenfield N, Fasman GT: Biochemistry 8:4180, 1969.
22. Chou PY, Fasman GD: Biochemistry 13:211, 1974.
23. Chou PY, Fasman GD: Biochemistry 13:222, 1974.
24. Chou PY, Fasman GD: Adv Enzymol 47:45, 1978.
25. Bewley TA, Levine HL, Wetzel R: Int J Peptide Protein Res 20:93, 1982.
26. Cell Tech Culture Product Division, Slough, UK.

2. Summary of Pre-clinical Data

P.P. TROTTA

Abstract

The data presented here summarize preclinical biological and biochemical data for highly purified, recombinant interferon (IFN) alpha-2 (Schering Corporation). These studies include (1) anti-tumor effects of IFN alpha-2 on malignant cells in culture and on human tumor xenografts in athymic nude mice; (2) anti-proliferative effects of IFN alpha-2 alone and in combination with cytotoxic drugs on cell lines and primary tumors in the human tumor clonogenic assay; (3) immunomodulation; and (4) evidence for the mediation of the biological activity of IFN alpha-2 through specific plasma membrane receptors. The significant results in each of these categories are summarized below.

In the human tumor xenograft model IFN alpha-2 has been shown to inhibit the growth of a human osteosarcoma, a human breast cancer and a human renal cell adenocarcinoma. Varying routes of administration were employed, including subcutaneous injection, intralesional administration and constant subcutaneous infusion for the three tumors, respectively. The data support that the human tumor xenograft model may be useful for predicting dose-response as well as the anti-tumor activity of alpha-2 and other IFN subtypes. In addition, studies with the renal cell adenocarcinoma indicate that combined therapy with IFN alpha-2 and difluoromethylornithine is more effective than single drug therapy. The mechanism by which IFN alpha-2 inhibits tumor cell growth appears to be related to a direct effect on tumor cell proliferation, rather than modulation of the mouse immune system.

A potent growth inhibitory effect of IFN alpha-2 was also observed in a number of normal and malignant human cell lines, including normal human amnion and breast cells, osteosarcoma, lymphoblastoid (Daudi), a T-cell lymphocytic leukemia (RPMI-8402) and a B-cell lymphocytic leukemia (BALM-2). The T-cell leukemia appeared to be markedly more sensitive than the B-cell leukemia. The human MOLT-3 T-cell lymphocytic leukemia, the murine P388 B-cell lymphocytic leukemia and a murine 239 Pu-induced osteogenic sarcoma were relatively insensitive.

Significant augmentation by IFN alpha-2 of the natural killer cytotoxicity of human peripheral blood monocyte-depleted lymphocytes against various hemopoietic cell lines and solid tumors has been observed. These data suggest that at least a part of the anti-tumor activity of IFN alpha-2 in man may be related to an indirect effect on the host immune system.

The first event in the expression of any biological activity of IFN appears to be the interaction with specific receptors on the cell surface. In an attempt to understand the biochemical basis for the various biological effects of IFN alpha-2, the binding of IFN alpha-2 to various human cell lines has been examined. Experiments employing I^{125}-labelled IFN alpha-2 suggest that IFN-sensitive cells contain a macromolecular receptor on the surface of the plasma membrane. Quantitative studies indicate ca. 102,000 IFN alpha-2 receptors per Daudi cell. A correlation will be sought between the number and/or affinity of IFN alpha-2 for its receptor and the anti-proliferative response of various malignant cells.

Introduction

The data presented below summarize aspects of the preclinical biological characterization of alpha-2 interferon (IFN alpha-2; Schering Corp.). This preparation is a greater than 98% purified alpha interferon subtype that has been cloned in *E. Coli.* The results presented here review *in vitro* and animal data in support of a direct anti-tumor activity as well as an indirect cytotoxic effect through modulation of the immune system. These studies have been divided among the following four groups: (1) anti-tumor effects on human tumor xenografts in the athymic nude mouse; (2) antiproliferative effects on malignant cells in culture; (3) augmentation of the NK activity of peripheral mononuclear cells against various hemopoietic cell lines; and (4) identification and characterization of a specific IFN alpha-2 receptor on the plasma membrane of normal and malignant mammalian cells. These experiments were performed by scientists of the Schering Corp. as well as by selected investigators at academic institutions. IFN alpha-2 employed in these studies was previously crystallized and re-dissolved in 20 mM sodium phosphate, pH 7.2. The preparation is stable in this buffer at -80°C; it is generally thawed and placed at 4°C just prior to use. Physico-chemical characterization of this IFN alpha subtype has been previously reported [1].

Results and discussion

Effects on human tumor xenografts in athymic nude mice

Osteosarcoma. In studies conducted by Dr. Douglas Kelsey of the University of Utah, a human osteosarcoma sensitive to IFN alpha-2 *in vitro* was implanted subcutaneously in athymic nude mice at sufficiently high cell numbers to produce a visible tumor in 7–10 days in all animals [2]. Measurements in three dimensions were performed at weekly intervals for quantitation of tumor growth. As shown in Table 1, intralesional administration of IFN alpha-2 at levels of 200,000 and 800,000 units per day for seven days resulted in a significant depression in the rate of growth of the tumors. Thus, for example, after six weeks post-inoculation, saline-treated mice demonstrated a mean tumor size of 1026 mm³, compared to 547 mm³ and 382 mm³ for the low and high dose IFN treatment, respectively. These data suggest that the nude mouse may represent a model for predicting dose-response. In other experiments (data not shown) it was established that intraperitoneal administration of IFN alpha-2 also results in a dose-dependent reduction in tumor size. Secondly, the data in Table 1 indicate that the acquisition of tumor is delayed by IFN alpha-2. Thus, one week following tumor inoculation 15 out of 15 mice developed tumors in the saline-treated group, compared to 9 out of 15 and 10 out of 15 in the low and high dose-treated group, respectively. In another study in which IFN alpha-2 was administered intralesionally at 800,000 units/day (Table 2), 13 of 15 tumors that were visible after one week were completely inhibited by the third week post-tumor inoculation. The reason for the apparently complete tumor regression in these experiments compared to the partial response described above at the same dose is at present unknown.

The osteosarcoma xenograft model was also employed to answer other questions related to dose-scheduling. Thus, for example, if therapy with 800,000 units/day was delayed to three days post-inoculation, no significant change in the

Table 1. Treatment of human osteosarcoma (Hos) tumors implanted in nude Balb/c mice with two doses of IFN alpha-2 (1)

	Mean tumor volume (mm³)					
Weeks post Hos inoculation	1	2	3	4	5	6
Saline-treated	12	34	101	214	529	1026
	(15/15)*	(15/15)	(15/15)	(15/15)	(15/15)	(15/15)
IFN-treated						
Low dose (2)	14	34	125	242	364	547
	(9/15)	(14/15)	(14/15)	(15/15)	(15/15)	(15/15)
High dose (3)	8	18	65	131	229	382
	(10/15)	(9/15)	(12/15)	(13/15)	(14/15)	(14/15)

* Numbers in parentheses represent the number of mice with tumors divided by the total number of mice.

(1) IFN alpha-2 is injected intralesionally 24 hours after subcutaneous tumor transplantation and continued daily for seven days.
(2) The dose was 200,000 IU/mouse.
(3) The dose was 800,000 IU/mouse.

Note: Data taken from Douglas K. Kelsey [2].

anti-tumor activity of IFN alpha-2 was observed compared to administration one day post-implantation. In addition, if animals that developed tumors after seven days of IFN treatment at 200,000 units/day were subsequently treated with 800,000 units, no effect on growth rate was observed. Thus, the latter results imply that a human tumor xenograft model for assessing the development of IFN resistance can be achieved. It is notable that a melanoma that was resistant to IFN alpha-2 *in vitro* was also resistant in this model.

In summary, these data suggest that the nude mouse model may represent an effective means for predicting clinical efficacy of IFN alpha-2 as well as for the evaluation of new interferon subtypes as they become available.

Renal cell adenocarcinoma. Dr. Timothy Ratliff and associates [3] treated a renal cell adenocarcinoma (JDF-1) (excised from a tumor in its eighth passage as a xenograft) with IFN alpha-2 by constant subcutaneous infusion. Two weeks following subcutaneous tumor implantation (mean tumor size: ca. 136 ± 14 mg), Alza minipumps were implanted subcutaneously that released 2×10^7 units IFN alpha-2 continuously over a two-week period. By implanting fresh minipumps at this time, IFN could be administered continuously for four weeks. In order to assess the potential for an interaction of IFN alpha-2 with alpha-difluoro-methylornithine (DFMO), a specific irreversible inhibitor of orinithine decarbo-xylase and a known inhibitor of mouse renal cell adenocarcinoma [4], a group of 20 mice received both DFMO in the drinking water and IFN alpha-2 by constant subcutaneous infusion, as described above. Another group of 20 animals was treated with DFMO alone in the drinking water; a control group (sham mini-pump implants) received buffer by constant infusion in lieu of IFN. As shown in Fig. 1, IFN alpha-2 alone as well as in combination with DFMO produced a significant ($p < .05$) reduction in tumor size. Control animals demonstrated a 5

Table 2. Treatment of human osteosarcoma (Hos) tumors implanted in nude Balb/c mice with IFN alpha-2 [1]

	Mean tumor volume (mm²)					
Weeks post Hos inoculation	1	2	3	4	5	6
Saline-treated	17	97	312	542	1222	1446
	(13/15)*	(15/15)	(15/15)	(15/15)	(15/15)	(15/15)
IFN-treated	9	2	0	0	0	0
	(13/15)	(2/15)	(0/15)	(0/15)	(0/15)	(0/15)

* Numbers in parentheses represent the number of mice with tumors divided by the total number of mice.

(1) IFN alpha-2 is injected intralesionally 24 hours after subcutaneous tumor transplantation at a dose of 800,000 units/day and continued daily for seven days.

Note: Data taken from D.K. Kelsey [2].

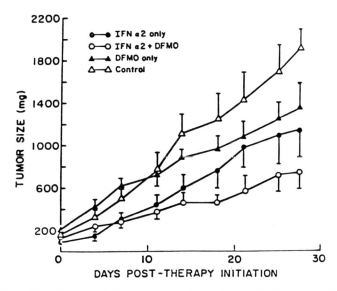

Figure 1. Effect of IFN alpha-2 and alpha-difluoromethylornithine (DFMO) alone or in combination on the growth of human renal cell adenocarcinoma xenografs in nude mice. JDF-1 tumors were implanted subcutaneously in the right posterior flank of 80 nude mice. Two weeks following tumor implantation four treatment groups (20 mice/group) were established: (1) Alza minipumps implanted subcutaneously and releasing 2×10^7 units per two weeks continuously; (2) DFMO in the drinking water as a 2% solution and minipumps containing buffer only; (3) DFMO in drinking water and minipumps containing IFN alpha-2; (4) minipumps containing buffer only (control). Tumor weights were estimated from measurements of length (L) and width (W) by the formule L × W ⅔.

day doubling time for tumor size, compared to 7 days for IFN alpha-2-treated, 5 days for DFMO-treated, and 14 days for DFMO plus IFN alpha-2. Thus, although IFN alpha-2 by itself was effective, the combination of the two drugs was more effective than either drug alone.

The additive interaction of DFMO and IFN alpha-2 as antitumor agents was further confirmed from mean tumor weights obtained at 28 days after surgical excision of the tumors (Table 3). The administration of IFN alpha-2 resulted in a statistically significant ($p < .05$) 37% reduction in tumor weight. Both drugs together resulted in a 58% reduction in tumor weight ($p < .0005$), which provided further support for a greater efficacy in the combination therapy. It is notable that IFN alpha-2 administered as a single agent appeared to be significantly more effective than DFMO alone.

Natural killer (NK) cytotoxicity utilizing ^{51}Cr-labelled YAC-1 cells was determined on splenocytes at the termination of the experiment at varying target to effector ratios. IFN alpha-2 resulted in no significant difference in NK activity, consistent with its known species specificity. DFMO, however, resulted in a greater than 50% reduction in this activity.

It is also notable that both IFN alpha-2 and DFMO alone as well as in combination resulted in significant reduction in spermidine levels and in the

Table 3. Treatment of human renal cell adenocarcinoma xenograft (JDF-1) implanted in nude mice with IFN alpha-2 and alpha-difluoromethylornithine (1).

Treatment	Tumor weight (wet wt., mg)		Inhibition	Statistical significance (2)
Sham implants	1484 ± 187	(520–2270) (3)	----	----
DFMO only	1106 ± 129	(730–1760)	25%	NS (4)
IFN alpha-2 only	941 ± 186	(20–1520)	37%	p .05
DFMO and IFN alpha-2	620 ± 109	(10–1420)	58%	p .0005

(1) IFN alpha-2 was administered by constant subcutaneous infusion (2×10^7 units in 0.2 ml per 2-week period). DFMO was present as a 2% solution in the drinking water. After 28 days animals were sacrificed by cervical dislocation, and tumors were excised and weighed.
(2) Statistical analysis by Student's test comparing experimental tumor weight to control (Sham Implants) tumor weight.
(3) Weight range, mg.
(4) NS, not significant.

Note: Data taken from W.D.W. Heston *et al* [3].

spermidine to spermine ratio. The reduction in the latter ratio appeared to be approximately additive for the two drugs together. Thus, effects on polyamine metabolism may provide a biochemical explanation for the apparently additive tumor effects.

Breast carcinoma. In experiments conducted by Dr. Taylor-Papadimitriou *et al* [3] nude mice implanted with a human mucoid breast carcinoma T1068 were treated with daily subcutaneous injections of IFN alpha-2 at doses of 50,000 and 200,000 units per day. In addition to weekly measurements of the two largest tumor diameters, tumors were excised and weighed at the end of the experiment. As shown in Table 4, IFN treatment for 23 or 35 days resulted in significant depression of tumor growth whether measured by weight or tumor size index (product of the two largest diameters). The differences between the control and treated groups were found to be highly statistically significant ($p < .003$ and $p < .001$ for Experiment A and B, respectively, at the higher dose level). These data provide further support for a direct antiproliferative effect of IFN alpha-2 on the tumor cells.

Antiproliferative effects

In studies performed at Southern Research Institute under the direction of Dr. Daniel Griswold (D. Griswold, unpubl.), IFN alpha-2 was tested for its effect on four different cultured lymphocytic cell lines: P388, a murine lymphocytic B-cell leukemia; MOLT-3 and RPMI-8402, two human T-cell lymphocytic leukemias;

Table 4. Treatment of a human breast carcinoma xenograft in the nude mouse with IFN alpha-2 [1].

Group	Daily dose IFN (units)	Tumor weights (g) Mean of each group of 5 mice (± S.D.)
Experiment A		
Control	–	1.08 ± 0.3
IFN alpha-2	5×10^4	1.18 ± 0.43
	2×10^5	0.39 ± 0.28
Experiment B		Tumor size index Mean of each group of 4 mice (± S.D.)
Control	–	1.96 ± 0.20
IFN alpha-2	5×10^4	1.65 ± 0.68
	2×10^5	0.94 ± 0.36

(1) In Experiment A, mice were treated with IFN for 35 days and in Experiment B, 23 days. The tumors were excised and weighed on the day of cessation of therapy in Experiment A. In Experiment B, the tumor size indices were measured from the two largest diameters after 23 days of therapy.

Note: Data taken from Taylor-Papadimitriou *et al* [5].

and BALM-2, a human B-cell lymphocytic leukemia. After 24 and 48 hours, cells were withdrawn from the control and test cultures, sedimented, washed, resuspended in appropriate medium and counted in a hemocytometer. Adriamycin was included as a positive control. As shown in Table 5, IFN alpha-2 at either 10^5 or 10^6 units/ml had no effect on the viability of proliferating cultured P388 cells, consistent with its species specificity, while adriamycin resulted in 88 and 97% growth inhibition at 24 and 48 h, respectively.

In contrast, incubation of RPMI-8402 cells with 10^3 units/ml resulted in ca. 100% growth inhibition after 24 h. Molt-3, the other human T-cell leukemic line, was also sensitive to interferon, but required 10^6 units/ml and a 48 h incubation to produce a 47% growth inhibition. The B-cell human leukemia BALM-2 was intermediate in sensitivity to growth inhibition, requiring 10^5 units/ml for a 67% growth inhibition, and 10^6 units/ml for complete inhibition. It is notable that all of these cell lines were highly sensitive to adriamycin. The biochemical basis for these differences in response is yet to be elucidated.

Dr. Sidney Smith of the Schering Corp. has examined the effect of IFN alpha-2 on the Daudi lymphoblastoid cell line (derived from Burkitt's lymphoma) cultured in RPMI-1640 medium containing 20% fetal calf serum. After both 3 and 6 days of growth, viability was determined by trypan blue dye exclusion, and cell count was evaluated with a hemocytometer. The data in Table 6 support that the

Table 5. Antiproliferative activity of IFN alpha-2 in human leukemia cells [1].

Cell line	IFN (units/ml)	% Inhibition of growth	
		24 h	48 h
Murine lymphocytic Leukemia P388	10^5	0	0
		88 (Adr) [2]	97 (Adr) [2]
Human T-cell leukemia			
Molt-3	10^5	0	0
	10^6	0	47
		100 (Adr) [2]	100 (Adr) [2]
RPMI-8402	10^3	100	82
	10^4	100	100
Human B-cell leukemia			
BALM-2	10^5	0	67
	10^6	100	100
		100 (Adr) [2]	100 (Adr) [2]

(1) After exposure to IFN for 24 or 48 hours, cells were sedimented, washed and counted in a hemocytometer. % growth inhibition is defined as:

$$\frac{1.0 - (N_t - N_o C)}{(N_c - N_o C)} \times 100$$

where N_t = cell density of the treated culture at 24 or 48 h.
N_c = cell density of the control culture at 24 or 48 h.
$N_o C$ = initial cell density prior to IFN or adriamycin.

(2) Adriamycin at a concentration of 0.2 μg/ml is the positive control.

Note: Data taken from D. Griswold, unpublished.

Table 6. Effect of IFN alpha-2 on the proliferation of Daudi cells (1).

IFN conc. (units/ml)	Number of viable cells/ml at Day 3 ($\times 10^6$)	% Inhibition	Number of viable cells/ml at Day 6 ($\times 10^6$)	% Inhibition (2)
0	1.79 ± 0.10	–	0.92 ± 0.04	–
1	1.29 ± 0.13	28	0.54 ± 0.07	41
10	0.73 ± 0.04	59	0.20 ± 0.03	78
100	0.48 ± 0.03	73	0.05 ± 0.02	95
1000	0.42 ± 0.04	77	0.03 ± 0.01	98

(1) Cells were counted 3 days after culture initiation, replenished with RPMI-1640 or IFN and counted again after 3 days (6 days after culture initiation). Data represent the mean (± S.D.) of 4 cultures.

(2) % Inhibition = 100 − $\dfrac{\text{Number of viable cells with IFN}}{\text{Number of viable cells without IFN}}$ × 100

Daudi cell line is highly sensitive to the addition of low concentrations of IFN alpha-2. Thus, for example, 10 units (equivalent to ca. 50 pg of protein) resulted in 59% and 78% inhibition at 3 and 6 days, respectively. It is significant that exposure to IFN alpha-2 for 3 days apparently did not result in the emergence of an IFN-resistant population. These data are consistent with evidence for specific IFN alpha-2 receptors on the Daudi cell, as described below.

Dr. Lowell Glasgow (L. Glasgow, unpubl.) of the University of Utah has compared the effect of IFN alpha-2 on human osteosarcoma, melanoma and amnion (WISH) cell lines (Table 7). The human osteosarcoma was the most sensitive of the three, exhibiting a 64% reduction in growth at 64 units/ml, compared to 12% and 14% reductions for the melanoma and amnion cell lines, respectively. It is of interest that the latter two lines were also observed to be relatively resistant to lymphoblastoid interferon (Wellcome Research Laboratories). The osteosarcoma employed in these studies was the same cell line from which the tumors in the nude mouse model described in Tables 1 and 2 were derived.

Immunoregulation

In preliminary studies conducted by Dr. Sidney Smith of the Schering Corporation, IFN alpha-2 was tested for its ability to augment the NK activity of peripheral mononuclear cells against ^{51}Cr-labelled K562 human myeloid cells as target. Target cells were incubated with varying ratios of effector cells, and the specific radioactivity released was quantitated, with an appropriate correction for spontaneous release of ^{51}Cr by the K562 cells. As shown in Table 8, a significant augmentation in lytic units per 10^7 effector cells was obtained at concentrations of IFN as low as 50 units/ml. On the basis of a mean control value of ca. 35 lytic

Table 7. Antiproliferative effect of IFN alpha-2 against human cell lines in vitro [1]

IFN alpha-2 conc. (units/ml)	Human osteosarcoma CPM	Human osteosarcoma % Anti-growth activity [2]	Human melanoma CPM	Human melanoma % Anti-growth activity [2]	Human amnion CPM	Human amnion % Anti-growth activity [2]
None	17,720	–	3,984	–	28,808	–
16,384	463	97.4%	2,150	46.0%	16,589	42.4%
4,096	734	95.9	2,323	41.7	18,344	36.3
1,024	1,261	92.9	3,090	22.4	21,809	24.3
256	3,055	82.8	3,509	11.9	25,273	12.3
64	6,328	64.3	3,496	12.2	24,653	14.4
16	10,734	39.4	3,680	7.6	25,042	13.1

(1) Growth was measured by incorporation of tritiated thymidine.
(2) Expressed as (1-Treated) (+ IFN) ÷ Control (− IFN)) × 100.

Table 8. Effect of IFN alpha-2 on the natural killer activity of peripheral mononuclear cells (1)

IFN conc. (units/ml)	Net increase in NK activity (mean lytic units + S.E.M.) (2)
50	43.3 ± 8.4
500	98.6 ± 26.3
1,000	91.2 ± 14.9
10,000	126.0 ± 49.5

(1) Data represent the mean value from 12 donors. ^{51}Cr-labelled K562 cells were used as targets. Target cells were incubated with effector cells at different ratios in a volume of 0.2 ml in microtiter plates. Per cent specific cytotoxicity is:

((E−S) (M−S)) × 100

where E = counts per minute released in the presence of effector

S = counts per minute released spontaneously in the absence of effector

M = counts per minute released after treating target cells with Triton X-100.

(2) A lytic unit is the number of effector cells yielding 30% cytotoxicity. It is expressed per 10^7 effector cells, and is determined by plotting the % radioactivity released versus log of the effector: target ratio.

units, the maximal fold stimulation was approximately 3.6 fold. This increase, which is comparable to the changes in NK activity that have been observed *in vivo* in response to biological response modifiers, would be expected to produce immunopotentiation of clinical relevance.

Dr. Chris D. Platsoucas [6] of the Memorial Sloan-Kettering Cancer Center has extended these studies to a variety of hemopoietic human tumor cell lines (Tables 9 and 10). The data shown in Table 10 are expressed as percent cytotoxicity as a function of the effector: target ratio for three individual donors. It is important to note that IFN alpha-2 can under specified conditions augment the NK activity of peripheral mononuclear leukocytes against each of these targets. The degree of augmentation, however, was found to be dependent on at least three factors: (1) The nature of the donor cells; (2) the nature of the target cell; and (3) the effector: target ratio. Thus, for example, at an effector:target ratio of 12.5:1, cells from donor 1 can be stimulated by IFN alpha-2 to lyse K562, Jurkat, HL60, CESS and DND cell lines, whereas stimulation of the other targets is not statistically significant. In contrast, the lysis of HL60, CESS and DND cannot be augmented by IFN alpha-2 if the cells from donor 2 are employed at the same effector:target ratio. It is also notable that certain cell lines appear to be resistant to lysis by NK cells, but that addition of IFN alpha-2 appears to confer a capacity for lysis. For example, it is only in the presence of IFN alpha-2 that donor 3 can lyse DND cells at effector: target ratios of 25:1 and 12:1. Occasionally, under certain conditions, IFN alpha-2 was observed to inhibit NK activity. In summary, the data strongly suggest that IFN alpha-2 is a potent stimulator of NK activity against a variety of targets, but the observed degree of stimulation *in vitro* is dependent on the conditions under which it is measured.

Table 9. Identification of cell lines

Lines	Origin
1. K562	Chronic myelogenous leukemia
2. Jurkat	T-cell acute lymphoblastic leukemia
3. HL60	Acute promyelocytic leukemia
4. U936	Histiocytic lymphoma
5. CESS	B-cell line EBV transformed (?)
6. HPB-ALL	T-cell acute lymphoblastic leukemia
7. DND	T-cell acute lymphoblastic leukemia
8. UGGL	Multiple myeloma

Table 10. Augmentation of natural killer cytotoxity of human peripheral blood mononucular leukocytes against targets from hemopoietic human tumor cell lines by IFN alpha-2 (2,000 units/ml). (1)

Targets	Treatment	Donor 1			Donor 2			Donor 3		
		50:1	25:1	12.5:1	50:1	25:1	12.5:1	50:1	25:1	12.5:1
1. K562	none	33.6±0.7	31.4±0.9	14.6±0.7	29.5±1.7	27.5±4.4	20.6±1.8	28.3±3.7	19.2±1.5	23.2±1.3
	IFN-α2	71.9±6.8	54.8±3.0	42.8±5.1	43.5±9.8	47.7±6.0	36.5±2.2	58.5±3.3	47.4±3.3	34.5±4.3
2. Jurkat	none	35.6±1.3	22.2±4.3	5.4±2.7	20.6±2.1	17.4±1.8	9.4±2.7	35.2±1.6	28.3±9.0	ND
	IFN-α2	72.0±2.6	71.5±4.2	64.4±0.9	85.0±10.7	71.9±1.5	ND	77.0±5.9	65.1±2.2	ND
3. HL60	none	5.1±3.9	3.7±3.0	0.05±0.0	17.5±4.5	9.4±3.7	8.5±2.0	8.2±3.3	0.9±1.2	1.5±2.2
	IFN-α2	29.7±10.0	17.5±4.5	8.5+2.0	28.2±2.8	19.3±2.9	10.8±8.6	37.1±1.5	22.5±4.5	16.7±4.1
4. U936	none	37.1±5.3	33.3±4.3	17.8±10.7	22.0±4.2	17.5±3.9	7.8±3.6	31.4±7.0	37.0±3.6	26.7±1.0
	IFN-α2	36.5±7.7	44.3±10.2	34.9±7.1	52.6±14.2	57.5±15.3	20.1±11.4	50.8±6.4	28.9±12.9	24.6±5.2
5. CESS	none	13.5±6.9	8.1±4.1	1.4±1.9	93.2±26.5	60.6±8.0	59.8±7.0	64.7±11.3	48.5±12.3	40.0±11.6
	IFN-α2	70.9±3.2	37.7±6.2	21.7±8.2	82.1±1.8	62.3±13.8	43.9±4.5	77.7±6.5	69.0±5.8	57.0±11.0
6. HPB-ALL	none	16.2±5.8	16.2±0.3	19.6±2.8	0.5±0.7	0±0	1.8±2.6	5.5±5.5	6.0±4.8	2.0±2.8
	IFN-α2	17.4±4.8	18.3±2.6	9.6±5.5	9.5±1.7	8.6±3.8	6.3±0.8	5.2±2.1	0±0	1.0±0.5
7. DND	none	32.7±3.8	12.0±1.7	2.1±3.0	21.2±1.5	8.2±6.7	0±0	8.9±1.3	0±0	0±0
	IFN-α2	86.8±8.2	68.8±22.5	58.9±3.5	12.4±8.8	6.1±4.5	0±0	28.1±1.7	22.8±1.6	9.8±1.4
8. UCGL	none	30.5±1.1	26.9±1.1	14.0±9.1	11.6±8.2	6.4±5.0	2.9±4.2	20.4±4.2	6.9±5.9	6.6±4.8
	IFN-α2	26.0±0.7	19.2±1.3	18.3±2.4	30.2±6.1	20.3±6.4	13.7±9.7	50.0±5.0	28.3±4.0	17.2±5.8

% Cytotoxicity

(1) Human peripheral blood mononuclear leukocytes were treated with 2000 u/ml of E. coli-derived IFN-α2 for 14 h at 37°C.

Note: Data taken from Higgins and Platsoucas [6].

Characterization of the IFN alpha-2 receptor

It is well established that in response to IFN treatment a number of gene products are induced, including protein kinase and (2'-5')-oligoadenylate synthetase, that have been postulated to be essential for the expression of antiviral and antiproliferative activity [7]. A number of early studies suggested that binding to the cell surface was the first event required for the expression of biological activity [8–10]. This binding presumably generates a signal whose ultimate target is probably the nucleus of the cell. In studies conducted in the laboratory of Dr. Sohan Gupta of the Memorial Sloan-Kettering Cancer Center, evidence has been obtained that the first event in the expression of the biological activity of IFN alpha-2 is a binding to specific, high affinity receptors [11]. Dr Gupta labelled IFN alpha-2 with ^{125}I employing solid phase lactoperoxidase iodination, followed by purification on Sephadex G-75 chromatography. As shown in Fig. 2, radiolabelled IFN alpha-2 was demonstrated to have specific binding to Daudi, WISH and SAOS-2 cell lines, each of which is highly sensitive to the antiproliferative effects of IFN alpha-2. Unlabelled IFN alpha-2 as well as natural leukocyte IFN and fibroblast IFN, but not IFN gamma, were able to prevent binding. Interestingly, the osteogenic sarcoma cell line U20S that is insensitive to IFN alpha-2 did not show evidence for the presence of specific binding (Fig. 2), thus suggesting either the absence of receptors or the presence of a much lower affinity class.

The binding of ^{125}I-IFN alpha-2 to Daudi cells was found to reach a saturation at 2,000 units/ml at either 37°C or 4°C (Fig. 3). At lower IFN concentrations, however, binding at 37°C was more efficient. Scatchard analysis of the data (Fig. 3, insets) indicated ca. 2,000 binding sites/cell with dissociation constants of 3×10^{-11} and 4.5×10^{-10} at 37°C and 4°C, respectively. It is notable that at 37°C a second, slightly lower affinity binding component was observed ($K_d = 3 \times 10^{-10}$ M), which is the main component observed at 4°C.

The technique employed for preliminary characterization of the IFN alpha-2 receptor was to incubate cells with radiolabelled IFN, followed by covalent cross-linking of the IFN alpha-2-receptor complex with either disuccinimidylsuberate, or dithiobis (succinimidyl propionate). Cross-linking with either agent yielded a radiolabelled complex with 150,000 molecular weight on SDS-PAGE. Similar results were obtained with WISH and SAOS-2 cells (both IFN alpha-2 sensitive) but not with the IFN-insensitive U20S. Furthermore, the complex could be immunoprecipitated with anti-IFN-alpha antibodies, providing further evidence that the 150,000 molecular weight species is an IFN-receptor complex.

It was also observed that pretreatment of the cells with trypsin abolished complex formation. Although neuraminidase treatment did not affect binding, the migration of the interferon-receptor complex on SDS-PAGE was altered. These data suggest that the receptor is a glycoprotein, at least in part.

Dr. Gupta and his colleagues also demonstrated that a portion of the bound ^{125}I-IFN alpha-2 becomes internalized by Daudi cells at 37°C [12]. This internalization was accompanied by a decline in the amount of the IFN-receptor complex detectable by cross-linking on the cell surface. In order to ascertain whether the internalized IFN was indeed present as a receptor complex, the cells were digested with trypsin to remove IFN bound to the cell surface, and the trypsin-resistant fraction was cross-linked. A complex of 150,000 was again detected on SDS-PAGE, consistent with the internalization of a IFN-receptor complex.

Dr. Baglioni and co-workers [13] have succeeded in the solubilization of the IFN alpha-2 receptor with detergent and the development of an assay for the

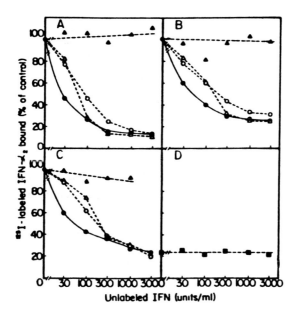

Figure 2. Binding of ^{125}I-labeled IFN alpha-2 to different human cell lines grown in culture tested in the absence or presence of increasing concentrations of unlabeled IFN alpha-2 (●), IFN alpha (leukocyte) (○), HuIFN-beta (△), or HuIFN-gamma (▲). A) Daudi cells; B) WISH cells; C) SAOS-2 osteogenic sarcoma; D) U20S osteogenic sarcoma. 100% binding represents 1180 cpm for A, 1120 cpm for B, and 600 cpm for C. With U20S cells (D), comparable binding was obtained (120–160 cpm) either in the absence or presence of increasing amounts of different unlabeled IFNs (alpha, beta or gamma). The 100% value with SAOS-2 cells (C) was therefore used to calculate the relative values shown in D. D is representative of all the sets with U20S.

solubilized protein based on ^{125}I-IFN binding. With the use of sucrose gradient centrifugation, an apparent molecular weight of 170,000 was estimated for the IFN-receptor complex, in general agreement with the data cited above. The calculated frictional ratio of 1.8, as well as the high partial specific volume (0.83) and apparent binding of large amounts of detergent, suggest that the IFN receptor on Daudi cells is a highly asymmetric and hydrophobic membrane protein.

Summary and conclusions

The data reviewed here summarize preclinical biochemical and biological evidence in support of a potent anti-tumor activity for IFN alpha-2. In the human tumor xenograft model IFN alpha-2 has been to inhibit the growth of a human osteosarcoma, a human breast cancer and a human renal cell adenocarcinoma. In view of the high species specificity of IFN alpha-2, it apparent that this result reflected a direct antiproliferative effect on the tumor cell rather than a host-mediated

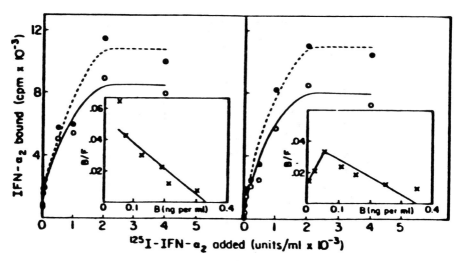

Figure 3. Saturation of [125] I-labeled IFN-alpha 2 binding to Daudi cells at 37° and 4°C. Cells (5 × 10⁶/ml) were incubated with increasing concentrations of ^{125}I-labeled IFN alpha-2 either at 37°C for 1 h (left) or at 4°C for 2 h (right), and the binding of labeled IFN to cells was quantitated by measurement of radioactivity after solubilization of cells in 0.5% SDS (●). Nonspecific binding of labeled IFN was determined in another parallel set of incubations in the presence of a 20-fold excess of unlabeled IFN alpha-2. The nonspecific binding was subtracted from total binding (●) to obtain specific, displaceable binding (○). The specific binding results from two experiments were averaged for the Scatchard plots (B/F, bound/free IFN concentration versus the amount of IFN bound) shown in the insets.

tumor rejection. This conclusion is supported by the failure of murine NK activity to be augmented by IFN alpha-2 administration, as well as by *in vitro* studies demonstrating a direct antiproliferative effect of IFN alpha-2 against a variety of normal and malignant cell lines. It is notable, however, that IFN alpha-2 produces significant *in vitro* augmentation of the natural killer cytotoxicity of human peripheral blood monocyte-depleted lymphocytes against a variety of hemopoietic cell lines. Thus, the anti-tumor effect of IFN alpha-2 in man most probably reflects a complex interaction of direct cytostatic and cytotoxic effects combined with an augmentation of host-mediated immune function. Regardless of the exact mechanism, however, receptor binding studies do suggest that the first event in these processes is binding to specific receptors on the cell membrane. It is an important area for future investigation to elucidate whether clinical response can be correlated with the nature of the IFN alpha-2 receptor either on the tumor cells or on the effector cells of the immune system involved in tumor cell lysis. Such studies should involve not only a determination of the number of such receptors, but also a quantitation of their affinity for IFN alpha-2 as well as elucidation of their chemical composition.

References

1. Nagabhushan TL, Surprenant H Le HV, Kosecki R, Levine A, Reichert P, Sharma B, Tsai H, Trotta P, Bausch Jr, Foster C, Gruber S, Hoogerheide J, Mercorelli S: Proc. of the Interferon Workshop, National Institutes of Health. In press.
2. Kelsey K: Treatment of a human osteosarcoma xenograft in Balb/c nude mice with IFN alpha-2. In prep.
3. Heston WDW, Fleischmann J, Tackett RE, Ratliff TL: Effects of alpha-difluoro-methylornithine and recombinant interferon alpha-2 on the growth of a human renal cell osteosarcoma xenograft in nude mice. Cancer Res, submitted.
4. Sunkara PS, Prakash NJ, Mayer GD, Sjoerdsma A: Tumor suppression with a combination of alpha-difluoromethylornithine and interferon. Science 219: 851-853, 1983.
5. Taylor-Papadimitriou J, Shearer M, Balkwill FR, Fantes KH: Effects of human IFN alpha-2 and human IFN alpha (Namalwa) on breast cancer cells grown in culture and as xenografts in the nude mouse. J. Interferon Res. 2 (4): 479-491, 1982.
6. Higgins JA, Platsoucas CD: Immunomodulatory functions of *E. coli* - derived human alpha interferons. American Association of Immunologists (75th Meeting), St. Louis, Mo., 1984.
7. Lengyel P: Biochemistry of interferons and their actions. Ann Rev of Biochem 51: 251-282, 1982.
8. Friedman RM: Interferon binding: The first step in establishment of antiviral activity. Science 156: 1760-1761, 1967.
9. Ankel H, Chany C, Galliot B, Chevalier MJ, Robert M: Antiviral activity of interferon covalently bound to sepharose. Proc Nat'l Acad Sci (USA) 70: 2360-2363, 1973.
10. Besanscon F, Ankel H: Binding of interferon to gangliosides. Nature 252: 478-480, 1976.
11. Joshi AR, Sarkar FH, Gupta SL: Interferon receptors. Cross-linking of human leukocyte interferon alpha-2 to its receptor on human cells. J Biol Chem 257: 13884-13887, 1982.
12. Sarkar FH, Gupta SL: Interferon receptor interaction: Internalization of interferon alpha-2 and modulation of its receptors on human cells. Eur J Biochem. In press.
13. Faltynek CR, Branca AA, McCandless S, Baglioni C: Characterization of an interferon receptor on human lymphoblastoid cells. Proc Nat'l Acad Sci (USA) 80: 3269-3273, 1983.

3. Synergy *In Vitro* and in Clinical Trials

C.E. WELANDER, H.B. MUSS, T.M. MORGAN,
P.P. TROTTA and R.J. SPIEGEL

Abstract

In vitro and *in vivo* studies have both shown synergistic cytotoxic effects of combined recombinant human interferon alpha-2 (rIFNα2) and standard chemotherapeutic drugs. The Human Tumor Clonogenic Assay has been used in this study to test the cytotoxic effects of rIFNα2 alone and in combination with eight cytotoxic agents. Schedule-dependent and concentration-related cytotoxicity of the individual drugs and combinations have been assessed. The greatest enhancement of cytotoxic activity is seen when rIFNα2 is used in combination with either doxorubicin (DoX), cis-platin, or vinblastine. Human tumor cell lines from carcinomas of the ovary, cervix, breast, kidney, and melanomas as well as biopsies from 14 patients have been tested with combinations of rIFNα2 and DoX. Results of these studies show that the maximal antiproliferative effect of rIFNα2 is related both to the concentration utilized as well as to prolonged duration of cell exposure; DoX cytotoxicity is maximized by prolonged cell exposure time to the drug.

Using clues from the *in vitro* data to design a clinical study, a protocol has been written, using sequential rIFNα2 and DoX to treat advanced solid tumors. Patients receive a simultaneous IM injection of 10 mil U/m^2 rIFNα2 plus 10 mil U/m^2 IV over 30 min. One-half hour later a two hour infusion of DoX (20 mg/m^2) is given. Three induction courses are administered one week apart, followed by a two week rest. Patients having stable disease or a clinical response are continued on maintenance therapy every two weeks. Seventy-five patients have been entered on study, including 16 ovarian, 13 cervical, 12 renal, 11 gastrointestinal, 5 breast, 4 lung carcinomas, 4 melanomas, 4 sarcomas, and 6 miscellaneous tumor types. Only one patient has been dropped from the study for Grade IV toxicity–temperature to 107°F with hypotension. Clinical responses to date have been seen in 5 patients with cervical, 4 ovarian, one pancreatic carcinoma and one sarcoma. Continued follow-up is in progress. The regimen is well tolerated and shows some clinical efficacy.

Introduction

Recombinant DNA technology has permitted the production of large quantities of purified human leukocyte interferon, providing now an opportunity to systematically study the antiproliferative effect of recombinant interferon alpha on tumor cells, both *in vitro* and *in vivo* [1]. Since the mechanisms are unknown by which recombinant interferon alpha induces cytotoxicity, attempts to study this effect *in vitro* and in clinical trials have been largely empiric.

One *in vitro* method of screening compounds for potential cytotoxic activity is the human tumor clonogenic assay (HTCA). This is described by Hamburger and Salmon, and has been widely used to survey a variety of human tumor types with both standard and investigational drugs [2–4]. Predictive correlations between HTCA results and patient responses to therapy have been acceptable, and are particularly accurate in predicting nonresponsiveness to a specific drug [5, 6]. Human tumor cells have been tested in the HTCA for sensitivity to various preparations of human leukocyte interferon [7–9]. Antiproliferative effects attributed to recombinant interferon alpha have been observed, quantitated in the HTCA as a reduction in tumor cell colony growth.

In vivo testing of recombinant interferon alpha has been done as Phase I–II clinical trials [10]. Since the theoretical mechanisms of action of recombinant interferon alpha may vary depending upon concentrations achieved in the host, the appropriate dose schedules, routes of administration, and frequency of treatment have been widely varied. Many clinical trials have attempted to identify the maximum tolerable doses and schedules that can be given to patients, thereby hoping to see maximum cytotoxic effects.

After testing recombinant interferon alpha as a single agent, the next logical step is to combine interferon with other cytotoxic drugs. Studies using human tumor xenografts in nude mice have shown synergistic antiproliferative effects of combined human interferon and standard chemotherapeutic agents [11]. In other *in vitro* studies using the HTCA, combinations of interferon with certain cytotoxic drugs have shown additive and occasionally synergistic combined effects [12, 13]. A broad *in vitro* screening study has been undertaken to determine whether cytotoxic drugs in combination with interferon can enhance the antiproliferative effects of each.

In this chapter, data are reported from HTCA studies of combined recominant interferon alpha-2 (rIFNα2) (Schering Corp., Kenilworth, N.J.) and eight cytotoxic agents, using six human tumor cell lines and tumor biopsy specimens from 14 patients. Analysis of the *in vitro* data has been made, looking for clues suggesting the optimal drug concentrations, scheduling, and sequencing necessary to maximize the overall cytotoxic effects. This information has then been used to design a treatment schema for a Phase I–II clinical trial of combined rIFNα2 and doxorubicin in patients with advanced malignancies. Preliminary results of this study are summarized in this chapter.

Methodology of *in vitro* studies of combined rIFNα2 and cytotoxic drugs

Tumor cells used for HTCA studies

Established cell lines derived from six human tumors have been used initially to screen varied concentrations of rIFNα2 and chemotherapeutic agents in combination. Cell lines were chosen because of the need for repeated testing of different drug schedules and sequencing schemata. These included a human ovarian carcinoma cell line (BG-1) (C.E. Welander, unpubl.), a human melanoma (SKMEL-28) [14], two cervical carcinomas (ME-180 [15] and CASKI [16]), a breast carcinoma (MCF-7) [17], and a renal cell carcinoma (CAKI-2) [18]. All cell lines were maintained as monolayer cultures, as described previously [19].

In addition, tumor biopsies from 14 patients were obtained, including carcinomas of the cervix (four patients), carcinomas of the ovary (four patients), endometrium (one patient), melanoma (one patient), brain (one patient), lung (two patients), and colon (one patient). Disaggregation techniques for these solid tumor specimens have been described previously [20].

Drugs used for the HTCA studies

Recombinant human leukocyte interferon alpha-2 (rIFNα2) was provided by the Schering Corporation (Kenilworth, New Jersey). The specific antiviral activity of this preparation is 1.7×10^8 IU/mg protein and is greater than 98% pure. In these studies, concentrations of rIFNα2 have been varied between 100 IU/ml and 10,000 IU/ml, attempting to correlate the HTCA concentrations with achievable plasma levels *in vivo* [21].

Eight cytotoxic agents, representing several mechanisms of action, were selected for the initial screening in combination with rIFNα2. The drugs included doxorubicin, cisplatin, 5-fluorouracil, methotrexate, vinblastine, bleomycin, triethylenethiophosphoramide and mitoxantrone. Concentrations tested of each drug were between 0.1 and 0.01 of the maximum achievable peak plasma level.

HTCA methodology

Single cell suspensions were prepared from either the monolayer cultures or from solid tumor biopsies as described previously [19, 20]. The drug exposure method used in the screening assays was either short-term (one hour exposure) incubation of cells with the drug prior to plating in agar, or long-term (continuous exposure), by incorporating the drug into the agar at the time of cell plating. Plating density of cells was adjusted to achieve approximately 200 tumor cell colonies per petri dish. This required 500,000 nucleated cells per 35 mm petri dish for the tumor biopsy specimens and between 25,000 and 50,000 cells for established cell lines. Details of the double layer agar culture system are similar to those described by Hamburger and Salmon [3]. Drug effects on cell growth were assessed quantitatively by colony counting, when aggregates of cells had reached a minimum size of 50 cells. Each drug concentration tested is plated in triplicate petri dishes, with six dishes for each untreated control.

Statistical methods of data evaluation

The HTCA data provide an objective endpoint for antiproliferative effects of drugs on tumor cell growth. Colony growth from cultures treated with drugs is compared to colony growth in untreated control cultures. The percentage colony survival is then compared between the various drugs tested, both alone and in combination. Details of the statistical methodology which permit evaluation of combined drug effect, have been described elsewhere [19, 22, 23]. The percentage colony survival when each drug is tested alone is multiplied together to obtain an expected colony survival. This is then compared to the observed colony survival when combinations of drugs are tested together in the assay. If the observed colony survival equals the expected, then additive drug effects are recorded; if the observed is less than the expected, this suggests a synergistic effect; if the observed is greater than the expected, this suggests some degree of drug antagonism.

Results of HTCA studies of combined rIFNα2 and cytotoxic drugs

Initial screening experiments with the six cell lines have been done, to determine the maximum degree of colony reduction in the HTCA by rIFNα2 alone, testing 100 IU and 10,000 IU with both one hour exposure and long-term continuous exposure. In the HTCA there was no reduction seen in colony growth to below 50% of control values with one hour exposure using any of the six cell lines when any concentration of rIFNα2 was used as a single agent. When rIFNα2 is tested in continuous exposure, it demonstrates antiproliferative effects only at the highest concentration tested (10,000 IU).

The cytotoxic activity of rIFNα2 and the eight chemotherapeutic agents was tested with cell line BG-1. Each experiment is done as a separate unit, with separate controls for untreated cells, for each drug tested alone, and for the combination of drugs tested together. Concentrations of rIFNα2 were screened, using 100 IU/ml and 10,000 IU/ml, each in sequential one hour exposures (rIFNα2 for one hour followed by drug for one hour prior to plating in agar) and in combined continuous exposures. The drugs showing the greatest degree of additive and synergistic effect are doxorubicin and cisplatin, the activities of which are summarized in Table 1.

Vinblastine shows a lesser degree of combined cytotoxic effect, best seen in the long-term continuous exposure assays.

Doxorubicin was selected as the drug to study further, and additional assays were done with the other five cell lines and with tumor biopsies from eight patients. Short-term (one hour) sequential exposure first to rIFNα2 followed doxorubicin were done, testing both 100 IU/ml and 10,000 IU/ml rIFNα2 concentrations with each. Synergistic cytotoxic effects were observed in two of the five cells lines (CASKI and SKMEL-28) and in one of eight patient samples (cervical cancer). Additive effects were seen in two of the other cell lines (CAKI-2 and ME-180) and in one additional patient biopsy sample (cervical cancer). Additional experiments using a reverse sequential cell exposure were done, exposing cell line BG-1 to doxorubicin followed by rIFNα2. In these studies the degree of colony reduction in the HTCA was equal to doxorubicin as a single agent, with no added effect from rIFNα2 seen.

Testing the clue that prolonged cell exposure time to rIFNα2 maximized cytotoxic effects, additional assays were done, using combined rIFNα2 and doxorubicin, each in long-term continuous exposure. Three cell lines (BG-1, SKMEL-28, ME-180) and five patient biopsy samples were used. Each of the three cell lines demonstrated synergy at both 100 IU/ml and 10,000 IU/ml concentrations of rIFNα2, with decreased percent colony survival seen at the higher concentration. Biopsies of one ovarian, one endometrial, and one cervical carcinoma showed additive combined cytotoxicity using the higher concentration of rIFNα2. The lung and colon carcinoma biopsy samples failed to show additive or synergistic effects.

Table 1. Fractional colony survival in HTCA experiments of rIFNα2 combined with doxorubin and cisplatin using cell line BG-1

rIFNα2 (IU/ml)	Exposure method	rIFNα2 alone	Expected colony survival	Observed colony survival	Combined effect	p value
Cisplatin concentration 0.25 mcg/ml						
100	1 hour	.92	.83	.52	synergistic	< .05
10,000	1 hour	.94	.85	.38	synergistic	< .05
100	continuous	.71	.50	.11	synergistic	< .01
10,000	continuous	.52	.37	.03	synergistic	< .01
Doxrubicin concentration 0.006 mcg/ml						
100	1 hour	.92	.68	.44	synergistic	< .05
10,000	1 hour	.94	.69	.47	synergistic	< .05
100	continuous	.71	.43	.012	synergistic	< .01
10,000	continuous	.52	.31	.02	synergistic	< .01

Conclusions of the *in vitro* studies

Review of these clonogenic assay data suggest that: (1) rIFNα2 as a single agent has some degree of cytotoxic activity demonstrable in the HTCA, but is limited to prolonged cell exposure time and to high rIFNα2 concentrations. (2) Additive and synergistic cytotoxic effects can be demonstrated in the HTCA when rIFNα2 is used in combination with doxorubicin, cisplatin, or vinblastine. (3) Maximal cytotoxic effect of combined rIFNα2 and doxorubicin will be seen when a schedule incorporating a long-term, high concentration of rIFNα2 and long-term exposure to doxorubicin is chosen.

Clinical Phase I–II trial of sequential human interferon alpha-2 and doxorubicin in advanced and recurrent malignancies

Design of clinical study

Using the information gained from the *in vitro* studies to design a clinical protocol, a Phase I–II trial using combined rIFNα2 and doxorubicin has been written. The schedule has incorporated the laboratory observations that interferon, when given to patients, should be given at high concentrations and over a prolonged time interval. Doxorubicin can be administered at lower concentrations, but will have maximal cytotoxic effect if the tumor cell exposure time can be prolonged. Logistical and practical considerations are also important in studies involving patient therapy in order to design outpatient treatment regimens when possible.

The schema for drug administration is as follows:

Time 0–10 million IU/m^2 rIFNα2 IM

then

10 million IU/m^2 rIFNα2 IV-infused over 30 minutes

½ hour–Complete IV infusion – wait 30 minutes

1 hour – 20 mg/m^2 doxorubicin IV infusion over 2 hours

3 hours – Complete doxorubicin infusion

The schedule of treatment courses has been designed to combine rIFNα2 and doxorubicin into a regimen which should not have excessive toxicity. Weekly doxorubicin administration schedules have been shown in clinical trials to be associated with less bone marrow toxicity and cumulative cardiac toxicity than larger doses given at three to four week intervals [24]. This study design has an "induction phase", giving three weekly courses of rIFNα2 and doxorubicin, followed by a two week rest. Response evaluation is then made, and patients with stable disease or any sign of clinical response are continued on "maintenance therapy", (in an identical schedule) given every two weeks. Patients having progressive disease at the response evaluation point are not continued on maintenance therapy. In schematic form, the treatment schedule is as follows:

Week 1 – rIFNα2 plus doxorubicin
Week 2 – rIFNα2 plus doxorubicin
Week 3 – rIFNα2 plus doxorubicin
2 week rest
Week 5 –Response evaluation
Maintenance therapy every two weeks

Therapy is continued until disease progression is observed or until the total cumulative doxorubicin dose reaches 550 mg/m².

Patients entered onto study

Eligible patients include those who have histologically confirmed malignant solid tumors which are advanced, recurrent, persistent, or metastatic. These patients must not be eligible for an appropriate higher priority protocol. All patients must have measurable or evaluable disease which can be followed for tumor response. Performance status must be $\geq$ 50% on the Karnofsky scale.

Of the first 75 patients entered onto the study, the tumor types are as follows:

Ovarian carcinomas – 16 patients
Cervical carcinomas – 13 patients
Renal carcinomas – 12 patients
Gastrointestinal – 11 patients
Breast carcinomas – 5 patients
Lung carcinomas – 4 patients
Melanomas – 4 patients
Sarcomas – 4 patients
Miscellaneous tumors – 6 patients

Toxicity of combined rIFNα2 and doxorubicin

Parameters monitored for toxicity of the regimen are those that have been classically associated with either rIFNα2 administration or doxorubicin therapy. These include myelosuppression, nausea and vomiting, neurotoxicity, fever, cardiac toxicity, and changes in performance status.

Of the first 14 patients who completed the three induction courses, toxicities are recorded in detail in Table 2. It is of note that bone marrow toxicity with weekly doxorubicin administration has been minimal. Reductions in doxorubicin concentrations from 20 mg/m² to 15 mg/m² have been required in only two of the first 14 patients and to 10 mg/m² in one additional patient due to hematologic toxicity.

Table 2. Clinical toxicity of combined rIFNα2 and doxorubicin (lowest recorded blood counts during 3 weekly induction courses).

Patient Number	WBC (mm³)	Granulocyte (mm³)	Platelet (mm³)
1	5,100	3,417	343,000
2	2,100	1,638	374,000
3	2,400	1,320	298,000
4	1,100	500	218,000
5	2,200	1,100	106,000
6	3,800	2,888	334,000
7	2,400	1,392	193,000
8	6,800	4,216	255,000
9	4,700	3,901	595,000
10	2,400	1,550	91,500
11	6,400	4,473	319,000
12	1,600	1,408	121,000
13	4,200	3,360	169,000
14	5,400	4,590	382,000

Transfusion – 1 patient for Hb. of 8 g.

Nausea and Vomiting:
Grade 1 – 3/14
Grade 2 – 8/14

Neurotoxicity:
Grade 2 – 1/14   Transient confusion with slurred speech

Fever:
Grade 1 – 11/14
Grade 2 – 0/14
Grade 3 – 3/14 (fever > 40.1°C.)

Cardiac toxicity – No decreases in left ventricular ejection fractions below baseline levels. No arrhythmias noted.

Baseline multiple gated acquisition (MUGA) scans have been done in all patients who have had $\geq$ 300 mg/m² prior doxorubicin therapy, and are repeated at each 50–60 mg/m² increments of doxorubicin. No decreases in left ventricular ejection fraction from baseline levels have been seen to date in any patient on study. The regimen is well tolerated and has not caused significant decreases in performance status. Outpatient administration of the regimen has been possible in many cases.

Clinical response evaluation to combined rIFNα2 and doxorubicin

Response criteria used in this study require complete disappearance of measurable tumor for a complete response; a partial response requires > 50% shrinkage of measurable tumor; stable disease is any tumor shrinkage less than 50% or no change in tumor size.

Progression of tumor implies > 25% increase in tumor size. It is still too early in the follow-up of this study to determine accurate response evaluation, as many patients are still undergoing treatment. The initial response evaluation following the induction phase of treatment and during a limited time on maintenance therapy has shown responses as summarized in Table 3. Additional time in follow-up beyond the first induction phase of therapy has been possible in some of the patients, and further clinical responses may still be observed. To this point

Table 3. Preliminary response evaluation of combined rIFNα2 and doxorubicin

Tumor type	No. evaluable patients	Clinical Response			
		Complete	Partial	Stable	Progression
Cervix	13	---	5	8	---
Ovary	16	---	4	9	3
Renal	11	---	---	8	3
Colon	4	---	---	1	3
Pancreas	3	---	1	1	1
Breast	2	---	---	2	---
Lung	3	---	---	3	---
Melanoma	4	---	---	1	3
Sarcomas	4	---	1	1	2
Miscellaneous	6	---	---	5	1

Table 4. Patients responding to combined rIFNα2 and doxorubicin regimen

Tumor type	Prior doxorubicin total dose (mg/m²)	Prior chemotherapy administered	Response to prior chemotherapy
Cervix	---	Bleomycin, Mitomycin-C	PR
Cervix	---	Cisplatin, Bleomycin	Stable
Cervix	---	---	---
Cervix	---	ICRF-159	Prog.
Cervix	---	---	---
Ovary	400	Cisplatin, Doxorubicin, Cyclophosphamide	CR
Ovary	---	5-Fluorouracil, Vinblastine	PR
Ovary	---	Cisplatin, Cyclosphosphamide	CR
Ovary	---	Melphalan, Cisplatin	CR
Pancreas	225	5-Fluorouracil, Doxorubicin, Mitomycin-C	Prog.
Sarcoma	195	5-Fluorouracil, Doxorubicin, Mitomycin-C	Prog.

in time, partial responses have been seen in 5/13 cervical, 4/16 ovarian, 1/3 pancreatic carcinomas, and 1/4 sarcomas. Additional background data regarding prior therapy and patient characteristics are provided in Table 4. Other evaluation parameters such as response duration, mean survival duration, and time on study cannot yet be determined.

Conclusions

In vitro data of HTCA studies suggest that rIFNα2 has some degree of antiproliferative activity when tested with human tumor cells. This property can be enhanced *in vitro* by combining rIFNα2 with doxorubicin, cisplatin, or vinblastine. A combination of rIFNα2 and doxorubicin in a clinical trial has been shown to be feasible, tolerable, and efficacious in the treatment of advanced human solid tumors. Further follow-up of the patients on this study is being done. Plans for additional clinical protocols using combinations of rIFNα2 and other cytotoxic agents are in progress.

References

1. Streuli M, Nagata S, Weissman C: At least three human type alpha interferons: structure of alpha-2. Science 209:1343-1347, 1980.
2. Hamburger AW, Salmon SE: Primary bioassay of human tumor stem cells. Science 197:461-463, 1977.
3. Hamburger AW, Salmon SE, Kim MB, *et al:* Direct cloning of human ovarian carcinoma cells in agar. Cancer Res 38:3438-3444, 1978.
4. Salmon SE, Meyskens FL Jr, Alberts DS, Soehnlen B, Young L: New drugs in ovarian cancer and malignant melanoma. In vitro phase II screening with the human tumor stem cell assay. Cancer Treat Rep. 65:1-12, 1981.
5. Von Hoff DD, Cowan J, Harris G, Reisdorf G: Human tumor cloning: feasibility and clinical correlations. Cancer Chemother Pharmacol 6:265-271, 1981.
6. Von Hoff DD, Clark GM, Stogdill BJ, *et al:* Prospective clinical trial of a human tumor cloning system. Cancer Res 43:1926-1931, 1983.
7. Epstein LB, Shen JT, Abelle JS, Reese CC: Sensitivity of human ovarian carcinoma cells to interferon and other antitumor agents as assessed by an in vitro semisolid agar technique. Ann NY Acad Sci 350:228-244, 1980.
8. Salmon SE, Durie BGM, Young L, Liu RM, Trown PW, Stebbing N: Effects of cloned human leukocyte interferons in the human tumor stem cell assay. J Clin Oncol 1:217-225, 1983.
9. Von Hoff DD, Gutterman J, Portnoy B, Coltman CA Jr: Activity of a human leukocyte interferon in a human tumor cloning system. Cancer Chemother Pharmcol 8:99-103, 1982.
10. Gutterman JU, Fine S, Quesada J, *et al:* Recombinant leukocyte a interferon: pharmacokinetics, single-dose tolerance, and biologic effects in cancer patients. Ann Int Med 96:549-556, 1982.
11. Balkwill FR, Moodie EM: Positive interactions between human interferon and cyclophosphami-

de or adriamycin in a human tumor model system. Cancer Res 44:904-908, 1984.

12. Aapro MS, Alberts DS, Salmon SE: Interaction of human leukocyte interferon with vinca alkaloids and other chemotherapeutic agents against human tumors in clonogenic assay. Cancer Chemother Pharmacol 10:161-166, 1983.

13. Yamamoto S, Tanaka H, Kanamori T, Nobuhara M, Namba M: In vitro studies on potentiation of cytotoxic effects of anticancer drugs by interferon on a human neoplastic cell line (HeLa). Cancer Letters 20:131-138, 1983.

14. Carey T, Takahashi T, Resnick LA, Oettgen HF, Old LJ: Cell surface antigens of human malignant melanoma: mixed hemadsorption assays for humoral immunity to cultured autologus melanoma cells. Proc Natl Acad Sci USA 73:3278-3282, 1976.

15. Sykes JA, Whitescarver J, Jernstrom P, Nolan JF: Some properties of a new epithelial cell line of human origin. J Natl Cancer Inst 45:107-122, 1970.

16. Pattillo RA, Hussa RO, Story MT, Ruckert ACF, Shalaby MR, Mattingly RF: Tumor antigen and human chorionic gonadotropin in CaSki cells: a new epidermoid cervical cancer cell line. Science 196:1456-1458, 1977.

17. Soule HD, Vasquez J, Long A, Albert S, Brennan M: A human cell line from a pleural effusion derived from a breast carcinoma. J Natl Cancer Inst 51:1409-1416, 1973.

18. Fogh J, Trempe G: New human tumor cell lines. In: Fogh J (ed), Human Tumor Cells In Vitro. New York: Plenum Press, 1975, pp. 115-159.

19. Welander CE, Morgan TM, Homesley HD, Trotta PP, Spiegel RJ: Combined recombinant human interferon alpha 2 and cytotoxic agents studied in the clonogenic assay. Submitted.

20. Welander CE, Homesley HD, Jobson VW: In vitro chemotherapy testing of gynecologic tumors: basis for planning therapy? Am J Obstet Gynecol 147:188-195, 1983.

21. Muss HB, Homesley HD, Rudnick SA, Plunkett S, *et al:* A phase I trial of recombinant leukocyte alpha 2 interferon in patients with advanced malignancy. Am J Clin Oncol: Cancer Clin Trials, in press.

22. Drewinko TL, Loo B, Brown B, Gottlieb JA, Freireich EJ: Combination chemotherapy in vitro with adriamycin. Observations of additive, antagonistic, and synergistic effects when used in the drug combinations on cultured human lymphoma cells. Cancer Biochem Biophys 1:187-195, 1976.

23. Momparler RL: In vitro systems for evaluation of combination chemotherapy. Pharmacol Ther 8:21-35, 1980.

24. Torti FM, Bristow MR, Howes AE, *et al:* Reduced cardiotoxicity of doxorubicin delivered on a weekly schedule. Ann Intern Med 99:745-749, 1983.

4. Discussion: Pre-Clinical Panel

D. KISNER and PARTICIPANTS

Dr. Kisner: I would like to start by making the observation that our first two speakers assiduously avoided discussing the issue of mechanism of action and I wonder if either one would care to comment on the mechanism(s) of action of alpha-2 interferon?

Dr. Trotta: Just about every mechanism that one could postulate for interferon has been postulated and there is some evidence for each of them. We know with certainty that there are genes that may be turned on by virtue of the binding of alpha-2 interferon to a cell surface receptor site. There may be genes that were not there previously, or expressed with low activity, that may be turned on by alpha-2. We know that this process is mediated by a specific receptor and that there must be some kind of a messenger acting between the binding of alpha-2 to a receptor and the turning on of these genes. Whether this messenger is the alpha-2 receptor complex, or whether there may be another messenger that we have not identified yet, we have not determined.

What the exact biochemical basis is for the expression of antiproliferative activity is not known. We could list all of the enzymes that have been implicated, including, for example, ornithine decarboxylase, which was the target of the studies mentioned earlier. They also include two 2,5-A-synthetase; there is activation of a protein kinase and there are effects on cyclic nucleotide levels. Just about every level of metabolism that one would venture to say could be affected is affected by alpha-2, extending from purine nucleotides to carbohydrate metabolism, to the metabolism of amino acids. It will be a great biochemical problem for the near future to resolve which of these mechanisms is operative in each of the biological activities that interferon expresses; I therefore leave that open for future biochemical investigation.

Dr. Kisner: Are there good clinical correlations with the NK data? Possibly Dr. Spiegel is going to tell us about this later. In fact, does the NK data hold up in clinical trials and is there a consistent effect on NK activity in patients given the material?

Dr. Trotta: I think Dr. Spiegel actually has data and I do not want to pre-empt his talk, so we will hear from him later.

Dr. Nagabhushan: Another subject that we have to address is that one has to develop animal models in order to determine the bioavailability of interferon in various tissues. We have to determine whether there is tumor permeability to interferon. This we cannot do with alpha-2 interferon in animal species because of the species specificity. Presently we are cloning and using mouse recombinant interferon in mice to investigate the bioavailability question. If we do such *in vivo* studies we will have a better idea of the bioavailability of the drug when it is used IV, IM or SC.

Dr. Kisner: Have there been any comparisons in biological systems between alpha-2 interferon and any of the native interferons in terms of relative activity?

Dr. Trotta: Certainly in terms of any of the parameters that I have mentioned, that is, stimulation of NK activity, anti-proliferative effects or anti-viral activity, there have been direct comparisons. The activities expressed are quite similar, although we find that if you look at the individual alpha sub-types that make up natural leukocyte interferon there are distinct differences within the alpha sub-type population. On the other hand, if you compare generally the mixture of interferon that is present in natural leukocyte interferon, the same trends hold, that is, biological activity is there in the same way that I have described and the specific activities per milligram of protein are approximately the same.

Dr. Nagabhushan: I would like to add that we were fortunate alpha-2 interferon is the major component of the leukocyte mixture. Again, with the evidence that we and others have, it does not appear that leukocyte interferon, or at least the major component of the mixture, is glycosylated, so that the recombinant DNA interferon, which is also not glycosylated, looks identical in that respect.

5. Phase I/II Clinical Trials

R.J. SPIEGEL

Abstract

Alpha interferon was one of the first recombinant DNA products available. It is now appropriate to review the experience with INTRON alpha-2 interferon to assess its activity and glean principles learned in testing this prototype recombinant DNA product that might be applicable to studies of future biologicals. INTRON was placed into nine separate Phase I trials, assessing effects of administration, schedule, and dose escalations. One hundred and sixty cancer patients and normal volunteers were involved. In addition to establishing maximum tolerated dose (MTD) and dose limiting toxicity these studies evaluated pharmacokinetics and immune modulation. Interferon produced toxicity that consisted largely of flu-like symptoms (fever, chills, lethargy) in over 90% of patients. Mild nausea and vomiting, mild hepatic enzyme elevation, and CNS toxicity were also problematic although rapidly reversible. Hematologic toxicity was also present although not considered dose limiting. Single doses up to 200×10^6 IU/M^2 IV could be given, although on a daily dosing schedule 50×10^6 IU/M^2 IV $\times$ 5d was the MTD. For continuous dosing 15–30×10^6 IU/M^2 S.C. TIW was the MTD. Phase I studies revealed INTRON to be safe with dose-related, predictable, and reversible toxicities which were predominately constitutional. In subsequent trials patients have received long-term treatment without any evidence of cumulative toxicity or intolerance. In most trials, greater than 90% of patients could be maintained on IFN therapy for long periods with appropriate dose and schedule adjustments being made.

Phase II studies have identified a number of promising leads for future pursuit and also a number of problem areas which will be important in the design and execution of future trials with other biologicals. In Phase II studies INTRON was not active by itself against most common solid adult malignancies: breast, colon, lung cancer. However, activity was seen in a variety of hemotologic malignancies including multiple myeloma, Hodgkin's and non-Hodgkin's lymphomas – particularly NML and NPDL where response rates may be >50%. Hairy cell leukemia appears to be peculiarly sensitive to alpha IFN. Kaposi's sarcoma patients also have a >50% response rate overall and greater than 85% of patients with limited disease may respond. There is also activity in some solid tumors such as malignant melanoma and renal cell carcinoma, although optimal doses and schedules have not yet been determined. In some of these trials responses occured after 4–6 months of treatment and many were remarkable for their completeness and durability.

In conducting interferon trials particular attention must be paid to effects of dose and schedule. Additionally, differences in patient population at entry can skew results and give rise to prematurely optimistic or pessimistic results. Interferon is tolerable but its toxicity is real. Expectations that other natural biologicals might be without toxicity are probably unrealistic. The prolonged time to response suggests that biologicals may require novel trial designs and be difficult to compare head to head with chemotherapy in which responses are expected promptly. Finally low response rates in some tumor types might belie the potential role of interferon or other biologicals. The quality of the responses seen, the potential for greater activity with a different dose schedule, and the potential for interfereon to work synergistically with other forms of therapy should all be considered prior to dismissing interferon's role in a particular tumor type.

Although the discovery of interferon is credited to Issacs and Lindemann in 1957, it was not until approximately 1981 and the availability of large quantities of highly purified interferon produced by recombinant DNA technology that conventional Phase I/II testing of interferon could begin. Alpha interferon was one of the first products produced by recombinant DNA technology and it is appropriate to review the Phase I/II experience with this compound not only to assess its own activity and toxicities but to glean principles learned in testing this prototype recombinant product that might be applicable to studies of future biologicals. Perhaps due to unfounded early expectations that interferon would in some way be a unique panacea for all malignancies, early clinical results have been greeted with disappointment and skepticism which are not justified. However, this reflects problems which are common to all new anticancer products and also special problems inherent to the testing of a prototype "biological" [1]. Among the special points to be considered in evaluating the results of interferon's early clinical trials are the following:

(1) Phase I/II clinical trials of new anticancer drugs are conventionally conducted in patients with advanced disease who have failed prior therapy. Thus we select a population with an expected poor prognosis and frequently with multiple drug resistance.

(2) Few antineoplastics give dramatic or clear-cut results at their earliest stage of testing. "Cures" are not to be expected and any levels of activity as defined by conventional Complete Responses or Partial Responses are taken as encouraging signs of a new drug's potential.

(3) Due to its species-specificity, preclinical studies are of limited relevance to clinical testing of interferons. This results in more unknowns at the time of first

testing in Phase I studies and leads to more extensive early clinical testing being required. This may add to delays before definitive results can be determined.

(4) The Phase I testing of biologicals requires novel trial designs which must choose between a cytotoxic versus a biological response modifier (BRM) model. In a cytotoxic model the optimal dose will be equivalent to the maximum tolerated dose (MTD), whereas the optimal biological response modifing dose may not necessarily be the MTD.

(5) Interferon may be most active in the adjuvant setting or with minimal tumor burden present. This prediction has been made since the advent of immunotherapy and some early trials are now supportive of this concept. This will be elaborated upon in this presentation.

(6) Finally, interferon and other biologicals may be very active in only some patients and it may be essential to evaluate not only the quantity but also the quality of responses seen. As an extreme example, monoclonal antibodies may eventually provide therapy that is 100% effective for only one patient [1]. Similarly, in early trials with interferon, certain patients have achieved complete responses of considerable duration whereas the overall response rate in given malignancies has not been high. If this result is confirmed in other studies then it might require a reassessment of our usual methods for screening new anticancer compounds.

With this background it is appropriate to look at the design and results of the early Phase I studies of INTRON to reach preliminary conclusions concerning best tolerated doses and schedules, predictable toxicity, and early indications of anti-tumor efficacy. INTRON was placed into nine separate Phase I trials to assess the effects of administration route, schedule, and a wide range of dose escalations. One hundred and sixty cancer patients as well as normal volunteers were involved in these studies. The schedules tested are outlined in Table 1 and show studies in which INTRON was administered by subcutaneous (s.c.), intramuscular (i.m.), or intravenous (i.v.), routes in a variety of schedules. It was given in a rising single dose with weekly escalations in a dose range from 1×10^6 to 1×10^8 IU. It was additionally given as a fixed daily dose for 28 days by each administration route, and it was given in a rising daily dose to determine the maximum dose that each patient could tolerate. Toxicity was primarily "flu-like symptoms", e.g., fever, chills, fatigue, myalgia, and arthralgia. Additionally some patients experienced mild nausea and vomiting (Table 2). Although these symptoms were present to some degree (mild to severe) in up to 90% of patients and were dose limiting, it is noteworthy that in all cases these side effects were dose-related and rapidly reversible. Additionally, in Phase II studies in which many patients have been dosed chronically for 6–12 months or longer, these types of constitutional side effects are non-cumulative and almost always become tolerable when patients' doses are titrated to their individual levels of tolerance (Table 3). Other side effects which appeared with lesser frequency included elevations of hepatic enzymes (SGOT and SGPT) and central nervous system

Table 1. INTRON Phase I trials

Single dose		
IM	×1	.01–100
Rising single dose		
IM	×1, q wk	1.0–100
IV	×1, q wk	1.0–100
IM	×1, q 72h	1.0–200
Fixed daily dose		
IM	qd × 28d	3–100
SC	qd × 28d	3–50
IV	qd × 28d	3–30
Rising daily dose		
IV	qd × 7d, qwk	3–100
IM	qd × 7d, qwk	3–100

Table 2. Non-hematology toxicity in INTRON Phase I trial: Single dose schedules.

	DOSE	
	≤10^7 IU*	>10^7 IU II**
	%	%
Fever	84	90
Chills/rigors	55	62
Fatigue/malaise/asthenia	30	52
Headache	36	56
Anorexia	29	49
Nausea/vomiting	30	62
Myalgia/arthralgia	25	22
Low back pain	13	14

* 176 patient exposures.
** 136 patient exposures.

toxicity, consisting of somnolence and occasional confusion. These were also dose-related and rapidly reversible upon cessation of interferon therapy. Table 3 shows these toxicities by severity and by their incidence in the earliest phases of treatment when patients' individual doses are being adjusted and during long-term maintenance. This table reveals that although most patients can be expected to experience some moderate to severe toxicity during their dose-adjustment phase, upon adequate titration of their individual dosages there are few symptoms that persist at a moderate or severe level. Table 4 shows a similar pattern observed in laboratory abnormalities. Mild hematologic toxicity occurs with interferon and it might be expected that if constitutional symptoms could be

Table 3. Non-hematologic toxicity in INTRON Phase II multiple myeloma trials/all toxicity grades (grade III or IV).

	Dose-adjustment		Maintenance	
Flu-like Sx	97%	(42%)	91%	(23%)
Dry mouth	27%	(1%)	16%	(0%)
Diarrhea	30%	(4%)	15%	(0%)
Somnolence	22%	(5%)	16%	(7%)
Confusion	14%	(1%)	5%	(4%)
Depression	9%	(4%)	13%	(2%)
Hypotension	7%	(1%)	2%	(0%)
SGOT	7%	(0%)	9%	(0%)

Table 4. Hematologic toxicity in INTRON multiple myeloma trials: Patients changing from WHO toxicity grade 0, 1 or 2 to grade 3 or 4.

	Dose-adjustment	%	Maintenance	%
HGB	11/37	29.7	9/27	33.3
WBC	22/39	56.4	8/25	32.0
Platelets	11/36	30.6	5/27	18.5
LDH	1/35	2.9	0/24	0.0
SGOT	3/42	7.1	0/30	0.0
SGPT	1/25	4.0	0/21	0.0
ALK PHOS	1/42	2.4	0/30	0.0

modulated, hematologic toxicity would prove dose limiting. Hematologic toxicity is rapidly reversible within 1–2 days after interferon treatment is discontinued and it has been suggested that this reflects delayed release of mature blood elements from the marrow, rather than myelotoxicity [2].

Maximum tolerated doses emerging from the Phase I studies are as follows: single doses up to 200×10^6 IU/M^2 IV can be given, although on a daily dosing schedule 50×10^6 IU/M^2 IV for a five day period is the MTD. For more continuous dosing, 15–30×10^6 IU/M^2 S.C. 3×/wk was the MTD. In summary, Phase I studies revealed INTRON to be safe with dose related, predictable, and reversible toxicities which were predominately constitutional. In subsequent trials patients have received long-term treatment without evidence of cumulative toxicity or intolerance. In most trials, greater than 90% of patients have been maintained on interferon therapy for long periods with appropriate dose and schedule adjustments being made.

48

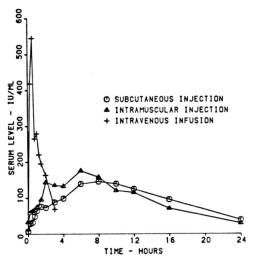

Figure 1. Mean serum level-time curves of interferon through 24 hours following single 10×10^6 IU doses of IFN-α_2 administered by three different parenteral routes.

In additional to establishing maximum tolerated doses and dose limiting toxicity, Phase I studies also evaluated pharmacokinetics of alpha-2 interferon (Fig. 1). Following i.v. infusion for 30 min, peak serum levels in the range of 500–600 IU/ML were obtained within 15–30 min. Following IV infusion, there is approximately a two hour half-life and serum levels return to baseline values by four hours. Conversely, both subcutaneous and intramuscular injection give similar pharmacokinetic profiles with peak levels reaching 100–200 IU/ML within four hours and sustained levels are seen for eight to twelve hours. Subcutaneous and intramuscular administration schedules therefore give a prolonged area-under-the-curve. Since *in vitro* models suggest that sustained exposure to interferon might be necessary to obtain maximum effects, most Phase II studies with INTRON have utilized a subcutaneous injection, usually in a 3×/wk schedule. In most of these studies patients have been instructed in subcutaneous injection and have been able to self-administer their interferon at home without difficulty.

Phase I studies were also designed to assay the immunologic activities of interferon administered in a variety of schedules and doses. Unfortunately, the results of these studies are largely inconclusive but the difficulties entailed in their design and execution may convey lessons for the study of future biologicals [1].

Initially, it should be recognized that at the present time our knowledge of the immune system remains rudimentary and only a small number of immunologic studies are available for quantitation when one wishes to examine a potential biological response modifier. In the case of INTRON the following studies were chosen as parameters: natural killer cell activity, antibody dependent cell cytotoxicities (ADCC), monocyte activity, lymphocyte subpopulation assays, and 2-5A-synthetase induction. The published literature reporting the clinical effects of interferon in a number of these areas is inconsistent. It is possible to find similarly designed studies given contradictory results of interferon's actions on any one of these parameters. This situation exists due to the heterogeneity of trial designs. One must be careful in reviewing these studies to note the type of interferon used, the dose, the schedule, and the sampling times when specimens were collected. The optimal time to look for immunological stimulation remains unknown. Finally, there is considerable heterogeneity in the way different centers perform their immunological assays with differences in target cells, sample processing techniques, etc. With all of these variables present, it is not surprising that results can be inconsistent [3]. It also remains unclear whether we are monitoring the proper parameters to truly assess underlying immune function. This remains an area where considerable development of trial design and standardization is necessary [4].

In Phase II studies INTRON has been administered to over 1,000 patients with a wide range of tumor types. In addition to following the conventional design of Phase II studies in which a new drug is administered to a predetermined number of patients with a variety of tumor types to see if it has true anti-tumor activity, we also need to determine whether differences in response rate might exist when interferon is given in different doses and schedules or to particular subgroups of patients. Our preliminary results indicate that interferon demonstrates both dose-dependency and schedule-dependency. Moreover, tumor size might play an important role in determining the expected response rates to be seen with interferon. For these reasons, low response rates in some tumor types might belie the potential role of interferon or other biologicals. The quality of the responses seen, the potential for greater activity with different doses and schedules, and the potential for interferon to work synergistically with other forms of therapy should all be considered prior to dismissing interferon's role in any particular tumor type.

References

1. Oldham RK: Biologicals: New horizons in pharmaceutical developments. J Biol Resp Mod 2:199–206, 1983.
2. Ernstoff MS, Kirkwood JM: Changes in the bone marrow of cancer patients treated with recombinant interferon alpha-2. Am J Med 76:593–596, 1984.
3. Sonnenfeld G: Contradictory results in interferon research. Surv Immunol Res 3:198–201, 1984.
4. Herberman RB, Thurman GB: Approach to the immunological monitoring of cancer patients treated with natural or recombinant interferon. J Biol Resp Mod 2:548–562, 1983.

6. Phase II Evaluation in Patients with Non-Hodgkin's Lymphoma The Old World Experience – An Interim Report

J. WAGSTAFF, D. CROWTHER, R.C.F. LEONARD,
J.F. SMYTH, H. HOST and N.C. GORIN

Abstract

This is a preliminary report of four phase II trials in the low grade non-Hodgkin's lymphomas (NHL) and two in high grade NHL. All the studies are being conducted with rDNA human alpha-2 interferon (IFN) (Schering-Plough 30500).

Low grade NHL

Two groups of studies are going on:
1. Two mega units per m^2 subcutaneously (SC) $\times$ 3 per week until disease progression or one year of therapy (Manchester and Paris).
2. One hundred mega units per m^2 intraveneously (IV) one day, then 2 mega units per m^2 SC $\times$ 3 per week from day 8. Cycles repeated at monthly intervals (Oslo and Edinburgh).

Schedule I

Twenty-nine patients entered. Eleven patients were diffuse well-differentiated lymphocytic (DWDL) and 18 have nodular histology. Twelve patients had received no previous chemo- or radio-therapy. Seven patients are still receiving IFN. There have been 1 CR and 10 PR (overall response rate 11/29 $\pm$ 38%). Eight of these are continuing in remission (duration 1 – 10+ months). The three relapses occurred at 2, 3 and 4 months. Six of 12 previously untreated patients responded (50%), compared with 5/17 previously treated (29%). Seven of 18 (39%) of the nodular NHL responded compared to 4/11 (36%) DWDL. Toxicity was mild and most patients tolerated therapy well.

Schedule II

Nine patients entered. Five were previously treated and three had DWDL histology. Two patients achieved PR (2/9 = 22%). Both are continuing in response at 2 and 6 months. One was previously untreated and both had nodular history. Toxicity in terms of influenzal symptoms and tiredness were more severe and debilitating on this schedule.

Conclusion

A substantial proportion of patients with low grade NHL still responded to IFN. Low dose continuous therapy is well tolerated over long periods. High dose therapy increases toxicity but does seem to produce a higher response rate.

High grade NHL

Two schedules have been used but the results will be considered together.
1. Twenty mega units per m^2 SC × 3 per week (Edinburgh).
2. Two hundred and fifty mega units per m^2 × 24 hour IV infusion monthly (Manchester).

Ten patients have been entered (8 Manchester, 2 Edinburgh). All were heavily pretreated. Nine had diffuse poorly differentiated lymphocytic NHL and one was lymphoblastic. There have been 3/10 PR (30%); of 2, 2 and 6+ months duration. The latter PR occurred on the continuous schedule. Toxicity on schedule I was severe and patients tended to progress between cycles suggesting that the more continuous therapy schedule might be more appropriate. However, patients need to be evaluated before firm conclusions regarding efficacy in high grade NHL can be made.

Introduction

The older methods for the production of Interferon (IFN) produced a preparation which was of low specific activity and of variable purity. This has made the interpretation of the early clinical trials difficult both in terms of comparing results between trials and within them [1]. The development of modern molecular biology has allowed the production of uniformly very pure IFNs for the first time, enabling the clinical evaluation of IFNs in a more scientific fashion.

A number of pre-clinical studies suggested that IFN might be active against lymphoid malignancies and clinical studies in small numbers of patients confirmed this early promise. A summary of these results is shown in Table 1 (for review see Horning, 1983).

In this paper we present the preliminary experience of several European groups with one of the new recombinant DNA human interferons, namely alpha-2 IFN (Schering-Plough 30500).

The results are summarised of four phase II trials of rDNA human alpha-2 IFN (Sch 30500) in the low grade Non-Hodgkin's Lymphomas (NHL) and two in high grade disease. The IFN was provided by the Schering-Plough Corporation. Formulated alpha-2 IFN, dissolved in phosphate buffered saline (pH 7.2), was freeze-dried in sterile vials and stored at 4°C. It was reconstituted immediately prior to injection by adding 1 ml of sterile pyrogen-free water.

Low grade NHL

Two regimes are being evaluated:
1. Two mega units/m^2 sub-cutaneously (SC) × 3 per week until disease progression or one year of therapy (Manchester and Paris). The Paris group treated two patients at 1 mega/m^2 × 3 per week. These latter patients will be included in the overall analysis of these low dose continuously treated patients.
2. One hundred mega units/m^2 intravenously (IV) on day 1 and then 2 mega units/m^2 × 3 per week from day 8. Cycles repeated at monthly intervals (Edinburgh & Oslo).

Eligible patients had a histologically confirmed diagnosis of one of the following Rappaport histological groups: Diffuse Well Differentiated Lymphocytic (DWDL), Nodular Poorly Differentiated Lymphocytic (NPDL), Nodular Mixed (NM), Nodular Histiocytic (NH). The study includes both previously untreated and treated patients with a performance status of 50% or more and a life expectancy of 4 months or more. Patients were excluded if they had a prior malignancy or had received IFN previously.

Twenty-nine patients have been treated with the first of these schedules and the characteristics of the patients are shown in Table 2. The overall response rates and the responses by sub-group are shown in Table 3. The median time to response was 2 months (range 1–6). Three patients have relapsed after 2, 3 and 4

Table 1. Summary of the results of leukocyte interferon in patients with NHL.

Histology	No. treated	Responses	Percent
Nodular lymphoma	38	17	45%
Diffuse well diff.	14	2	14%
Diffuse histiocytic	15	0	–

months and the response duration of the patients continuing in remission is between 1 and 10 months.

Toxicity has been mild. Patients invariably developed an influenza-like syndrome after the first few injections. This consisted of fever, shivering, myalgia and headache lasting for up to 12 hours. However, tachyphylaxis developed and by the end of the first week the majority of patients had no side effects or very mild ones. Some patients developed increased tiredness but in general this did not interfere with their lives. Many patients were able to give the IFN to themselves thus minimising the interruption to their daily activities. Haematologic toxicity was mild with the white blood count increasing by one WHO grade (median WBC = 3.3 (1.0–9.7)). No patient had treatment suspended or delayed because of haematological toxicity. Platelet counts were less affected than WBC. There was no clinically significant alteration of liver function. Approximately 10% of patients developed non-pruritic, non-tender erythema at the injection sites which

Table 2. Characteristics of patients with low grade NHL treated in Manchester and Paris.

Age	Median 58 yrs.	(37–72)
Performance status	Median 90%	(60–90)
Stage	III	7
	IV	22
Symptoms	A	24
	B	5
Prior CT/XRT	No	12
	Yes	17
Refractory to CT		6
Histology		
Diffuse well diff. lymphocytic		11
Nodular histiocytic		2
Nodular mixed		5
Nodular poorly		
diff. lymphocytic		11

Table 3. Response to alpha 2 IFN by subgroup.

	Responses	Number	Percent
Histology			
Diffuse	4	11	36%
Nodular	7	18	39%
Prior treatment			
None	6	12	50%
More than 3	4	12	33%
Months after			
Refractory	1	5	20%

took 3 to 4 days to resolve. No patient had to stop therapy because of this. Three patients in Manchester developed reactivation of latent peri-oral Herpes simplex infection.

Nine patients have been treated with the second schedule (Edinburgh/Oslo). Two patients have achieved partial responses, both of which are continuing at 2 and 6 months. One patient was previously untreated and both had nodular histologies. Toxicity of this schedule was more severe with a more dramatic influenzal syndrome and more profound tiredness and lethargy. Haematological toxicity was not however a clinical problem.

In summary there is an overall response rate of 13 of 38 patients treated (1 CR & 8 PR = 34%). The response rate at the present time is higher in those treated with schedule one (38% vs 22%) and the toxicity is less. Responses occur more commonly in previously untreated patients (50%) versus 33% in those who have not received chemotherapy for 3 months and least often in those who are refractory (20%). There does not as yet seem to be a different response rate for any particular histological group.

High grade NHL

Two schedules have been used:
1. Manchester: 250 mega units/m^2 IV as a twenty-four hour infusion repeated at 3 to 4 weekly intervals until disease progression.
2. Edinburgh: 20 mega units/m^2 SC × 3 per week until disease progression.

Ten patients have been entered (8 Manchester and 2 Edinburgh). Nine had diffuse poorly differentiated lymphocytic and 1 lymphoblastic lymphoma. All the patients were heavily pre-treated. Three patients have achieved PR of 2, 2 & 6+ months' duration. The latter patient was treated on schedule two. Two further patients had a 50% regression of measurable disease on schedule one, but the disease progressed within one month.

Toxicity of schedule one was severe. A profound influenzal syndrome associated with severe rigors, nausea and vomiting occurred during the infusion. The patients became anorexic, tired and lethargic for 1 to 2 weeks after the treatments. They found it increasingly hard to continue therapy. The second schedule was better tolerated but toxicity was still moderately severe. Haematological toxicity was not dose limiting.

High grade lymphomas do seem to respond to IFN given at these doses and in this way but toxicity is severe. The fact that patients tend to relapse between courses suggests that the more continuous treatment of schedule two might be more appropriate. These conclusions must remain guarded until more patients with this disease are evaluated.

References

1. Alexanian R, Gutterman J, Levy H: Interferon treatment for multiple myeloma. Clin Haemato II:211, 1982.
2. Horning S: Lymphoma. In Interferon in Cancer, Sikora K (ed). Plenum Press, New York & London, 1983, p 77.

7. High and Low Dose Treatment for High and Low Grade Non-Hodgkin's Lymphoma

R.D. LEAVITT, S. KAPLAN, E. BONNEM, M. GRIMM,
H. OZER, C. PORTLOCK, V. RATANATHARATHORN,
C. KARANES, J. ULTMANN and S. RUDNICK

Abstract

Forty-nine patients with non-Hodgkin's lymphoma were treated with recombinant alpha-2 interferon (Schering Corporation Intron) at five cooperating institutions in the United States and are evaluable for response. Results from ten evaluable patients with low grade histology and six evaluable patients with high grade histology treated at the University of Maryland Cancer Center are reported in detail. The results of response to interferon treatment in patients with low grade and high grade histologies are reported from the other institutions. Patients with low grade histology received interferon 10 MU/m^2 subcutaneously, three times weekly, for at least six months or for an additional two months following maximal response. In the group's experience, 45% of evaluable patients with low grade lymphomas had complete or partial responses with a median duration of seven months. Response in the low grade lymphomas was seen only in the nodular histologies. One patient with hairy cell leukemia who relapsed after previous splenectomy, radiation therapy, and chemotherapy, achieved partial remission and continues treatment. In the high grade lymphomas, the overall response rate in heavily pretreated patients was 13%. The toxicities were substantial. Many patients are not evaluable for response because of early cessation of treatment, either from advancing disease or from interferon toxicity. Even when interferon was admininistered at full dose and without delay in treatment cycles, there was frequently rapid progression of disease. However, complete response was seen in three patients with diffuse undifferentiated lymphoma with T-cell markers, diffuse large cell lymphoma, and diffuse poorly differentiated lymphocytic lymphoma. Further study is necessary to determine if certain histologic subtypes or cell surface marker phenotypes of high grade lymphoma are responsive to interferon treatment.

Introduction

The alpha interferons are natural biological proteins with potent ability to regulate a number of biological responses. Early clinical trials in man were conducted using material isolated from the buffy coat of blood donations. Obtaining even small quantities of "buffy coat" interferon for clinical trials in man required processing huge volumes of donated blood. The material obtained was of low purity, with typically 1-2% of the protein content present as interferon. Moreover, there were other biologically active agents present including endotoxin and leukocyte pyrogen. It was not possible to know which of the toxicities and actions of "interferon" were actually attributable to the contaminants. Alpha interferon of increased purity has subsequently been produced from human cells in tissue culture. The purity of lymphoblastoid interferon is typically more than 50% of protein present as interferon. Large-scale trials of interferon in man, however, were initially spurred by the development of recombinant leukocyte interferons. This allowed the large-scale production of a single molecular species of alpha interferon in *E. coli*. Subsequent purification procedures produce a product in which virtually all protein present is a single species of alpha interferon. Other material which may be present, such as antibiotics used in the purification process or bacterial products such as endotoxin, are reduced to either negligible or undetectable levels.

Human clinical trials of alpha interferons have been concentrated in two groups of patients – those with viral infections and those with advanced malignancy. Early clinical trials with partially pure interferons have included patients with untreated and relapsed lymphomas. Invariably, lymphomas have been among the most frequent types of malignancy to show objective evidence of antitumor response to interferon therapy [9, 19]. Treatment of non-Hodgkin's lymphoma with interferon has shown greater promise in the nodular type than in the diffuse form. One study showed an effect in three of three patients with nodular type [9], while in another, regression was achieved in six of eight evaluable patients, two of whom had a complete regression [10]. Early Phase I trials with two recombinant human alpha interferon preparations, conducted at the University of Maryland Cancer Center and other institutions, have shown frequent responses in patients with lymphomas [11-14]. It is not possible to assess the precise activity of interferon in lymphoma from the results of these Phase I toxicity tests. In both the Phase I testing of recombinant alpha interferon and in previous studies with partially pure interferon, patients included have been heterogeneous in lymphoma histology, extent of disease, and previous treatment. Evaluation criteria were frequently not rigorous. Patients have been treated with only a narrow range of dosages and schedules because of the limited availability and great expense of material. When using partially pure interferon preparations, it was unclear if antitumor effects were responses to interferon or other contaminating substances.

The collected experience of treatment of lymphomas with recombinant or natural interferon has been almost exclusively in the lymphomas of low-grade histology, for several reasons. Chronic lymphocytic leukemia and diffuse-well differentiated lymphoma (International Working Formulation-A), nodular poorly differentiated lymphocytic lymphoma (IWF-B) and nodular mixed lymphoma (IWF-C) frequently follow a more indolent clinical course, during which it is possible to conduct clinical trials with new agents. Delay of conventional therapy need not be detrimental to patient care in this setting. In usual practice, selected patients are frequently closely observed without treatment. Early treatment, even in the presence of active lymphoma, may not improve clinical outcome. In the less common nodular histiocytic lymphoma (IWF-D), early treatment may provide the opportunity for long-term, disease-free survival. Untreated patients with this histology may not be appropriate for inclusion in trials of new investigational agents because they may derive more benefit from conventional treatment. Experience with treatment of relapsed nodular histiocytic lymphoma is limited because the histology is less common and because there is a frequent change to diffuse histiocytic lymphoma (IWF-G or IWF-H) and more aggressive clinical course at the time of relapse.

The experience with interferon treatment of high grade lymphomas is limited. Patients with diffuse mixed lymphomas (IWF-F), diffuse histiocytic lymphoma (IWF-G or IWF-H), lymphoblastic lymphoma (IWF-I) and diffuse undifferentiated lymphoma (IWF-J) are widely recognized as having the opportunity for long-term, disease-free survival and possible cure following conventional treatment. Untreated patients with these high grade histologies are therefore not candidates for initial treatment with investigational new agents. At the time of relapse these patients are frequently not appropriate candidates for conventional Phase I of Phase II trials. Relapsed disease may be rapidly progressive, requiring prompt treatment with agents of known efficacy. Patient performance status, marrow reserve, and expected length of survival may also be insufficient to allow an adequate evaluation of the efficacy of a new agent. Nevertheless, there is a need for new therapies for relapsed high grade lymphomas. Almost invariably, patients who relapse will eventually succumb to their lymphoma or complications of its treatment. Moreover, survival following relapse is frequently short. Resistance to conventional agents is often present at relapse or develops shortly thereafter. The intensity of treatment is further limited by decreased bone marrow reserve, as a result of both the cumulative effects of lymphoma treatment and the frequent involvement of marrow with lymphoma at the time of relapse. This may make treatment with full doses of potentially effective agents impossible. In patients with diffuse poorly differentiated lymphocytic lymphoma (IWF-E), the potential for prolonged disease-free survival following chemotherapy probably does not exist for most patients. Early relapse and progressive disease is frequent. No recent advance in therapy has much improved the prognosis of these patients.

The experience and treatment of high grade lymphomas with interferon has been limited. Most untreated patients with high grade lymphoma have been appropriately treated with conventional agents. At the time of relapse, even effective palliation has required that there be a chance for early response. Treatment of low grade lymphomas with lower doses of interferon gives responses which are frequently delayed many weeks. Such a delay would effectively preclude the chance for response in a patient with a rapidly progressive lymphoma. In fact, in the few reported cases of treatment of high grade lymphoma with relatively low doses of natural alpha interferon, patients have had rapidly progressive disease and no useful antitumor responses have been observed [9, 10].

Phase I trials of toxicity and tolerance to alpha interferon have used a wide variety of doses and schedules. The toxicities experienced with two recombinant DNA-produced interferons and one lymphoblastoid product are similar [11–14]. Low to moderate doses of interferon, up to 10 million units/m² average daily dose, by subcutaneous, intramuscular, or intravenous injection are well tolerated, whether given three times weekly, daily, or twice daily. Observed toxicities include mild, reversible myelosuppression, hepatotoxicity, and fatigue. All patients experience a flu-like syndrome at the initiation of therapy. For most patients there is rapid tolerance established to this side effect. Many patients will tolerate treatment with lower dose interferon for prolonged periods of time. However, at the higher doses fatigue, malaise, anorexia and weight loss may become intolerable, requiring either the cessation of treatment or marked reduction of dosage. At higher doses of interferon, side effects are more likely to be dose limiting. At doses above an average of 50 million units daily, neutropenia and elevation of hepatic transaminases are frequent. These side effects are rapidly reversible on cessation of treatment. However, profound fatigue, malaise and even mental confusion prevent prolonged treatment with high doses.

High doses of interferon, however, can be tolerated for short periods of time. Doses of 30 to 50 ml/m² daily for 5 days can be given either as a continuous intravenous infusion or as daily 30 minute infusions with acceptable toxicity. Although flu-like symptoms and fatigue may be profound , recovery allows the repetition of this schedule every 2 to 3 weeks. Myelosuppression is more severe than with lower doses but is usually rapidly reversible. With a 5 day course of treatment, hepatotoxicity is less frequent and less severe than with more prolonged administration.

The work reported here was undertaken to determine the level of efficacy of interferon in the treatment of low grade and high grade lymphomas. It was felt that the true value of therapy with a new agent with known antilymphoma activity should include assessment in patients who are previously untreated or who have not been heavily previously treated. This is possible in selected patients with newly diagnosed or relapsed low grade lymphomas who might otherwise be safely managed under careful observation alone. Except in diffuse poorly differentiated lymphocytic lymphoma, investigational therapy of high grade lymphomas must necessarily be delayed until the time of relapse, when conventional therapy is not known to produce a lasting benefit.

Patients with low grade lymphoma were treated with a less intense dose and schedule. The expected clinical course is such that patients will derive benefit from a clinical response, even if the response is delayed for several weeks. Moreover, responses may improve gradually. Prolonged treatment may be necessary in order to derive maximum clinical benefit. Therefore, a potentially beneficial but less intensive regimen will permit long-term drug administration with acceptable toxicity in these patients.

In high grade lymphomas more intense treatment was given, since beneficial response may need to be obtained promptly. Preliminary experience from other clinical trials in a limited number of patients also suggests that high grade lymphomas are not as sensitive to the antitumor effects of interferon as are lymphomas of low grade histology. Therefore, a trial to determine the potential antitumor activity of alpha interferon in high grade lymphomas was designed to include high doses given in a short course. This might also allow the opportunity to assess potential antitumor activity in a short period of time. Patients with early progressive disease would not be expected to achieve a better response with more prolonged therapy. These patients would then be able to receive subsequent treatment with conventional agents that may have some palliative benefit.

This paper reports the combined experience of several centers in the treatment of non-Hodgkin's lymphoma with recombinant alpha-2 interferon (Schering Corp. Intron). Patients with lymphoma of low grade histology, either at presentation or at relapse, were treated with lower dose interferon. Patients with relapsed or refractory high grade lymphoma, or previously untreated diffuse poorly differentiated lymphocytic lymphoma, were treated with intermittent, high doses of intravenous interferon. Patients with low grade histology had a high rate of response. Treatment of high grade lymphomas was accompanied by a higher rate of complications, poor treatment tolerance, and a low rate of response. There is no evidence that any one histology of high grade lymphoma is more responsive to interferon treatment than any other histology.

Methods and materials

Interferon preparation

Recombinant leukocyte alpha-2 interferon (Schering Corp., Intron) was supplied as a lyophilized powder containing 10 million or 50 million international units in a vial to be reconstituted to a total volume of 1ml with sterile water. The lyophilized powder was stored at 4°C. Reconstituted material was stored refrigerated and used within 24 hours. Patients receiving subcutaneous interferon were given 2 weeks' supply of drug for home use, where they daily reconstitued material for self injection. During the course of the study the recombinant interferon was prepared by two procedures, MISH and KMAC. The MISH preparation contained trace amounts of ampicillin used in the isolation procedure. A single patient with a history of cutaneous hypersensitivity to penicillin developed a macular skin rash while taking the MISH preparation. This disappeared following discontinuation of treatment and did not reappear when the patient was retreated with the KMAC preparation.

Toxicity measurements

Toxicities were graded according to the WHO recommendations for grading of acute and sub-acute toxicity. Dosage was adjusted for grade III or grade IV toxicity.

Evaluation criteria

Before treatment all patients had chest x-ray, bilateral bone marrow aspirates and biopsies, serum protein electrophoresis, and standard hematological and chemical screening including coagulation studies. Urinalysis and electrocardiogram were also obtained prior to treatment. Additional studies were obtained as necessary to measure disease involvement or as clinically indicated. Most patients had computerized tomography (CT) of abdomen, liver and pelvis. Additional studies frequently included CT scan of the thorax, gallium scan, contrast x-rays of upper G.I. tract and small bowel, bone scan, bone x-rays, and CT scan of the brain. Studies in this group were repeated as clinically indicated and no less frequently than every 8 to 12 weeks.

Patient selection

Patients with non-Hodgkin's lymphoma of high or low grade histology were entered into study between June 1982 and February, 1984. Diagnostic histological material was reviewed by an experienced hematopathologist. Patients were considered to have low grade histologies if they were classified in the International Working Formulation as A, B, or C. Patients with histologic types D – J were classified as high grade lymphoma. Patients with low grade histology were either previously untreated or had relapsed after radiotherapy or chemotherapy. All patients had stage III or IV disease, a performance status better than two (ECOG five grade scale), and had an estimated life expectancy of at least six weeks. All had measurable disease outside of any previously radiated areas. Repeat biopsy of involved tissue was done within four weeks of therapy unless the biopsy would have required a major surgical procedure. All patients were at least 28 days from any prior therapy and had recovered from any previous acute drug toxicity. All patients had adequate marrow reserve (granulocytes greater than 1500/mm^3, hemoglobin greater than 10 dl, and platelets greater than 100,000/mm³), unless the abnormalities were due to documented infiltration of the marrow by lymphoma. All patients had normal renal function (creatinine less than 1.9) and hepatic function (SGOT less than two times the upper limit of normal), unless the abnormalities were judged to be due to the presence of lymphoma. Patients with high grade lymphoma were eligible for study if they had relapsed histologies, IWFD-I or newly diagnosed or relapsed histology IWF-E. All patients had clearly measurable disease, performance status better than 2, and an expected six week survival. No patient with either high or low grade histology was eligible for study if there was central nervous system disease, major surgery within one month of treatment, other malignancy, previous treatment with another interferon preparation, or the presence of an active infection. Patients were excluded from study if they had a history of recent myocardial infarction, congestive heart failure, or severe hypertension or previous treatment with anticoagulant drugs.

Interferon dose and schedule

Patients with low grade lymphoma were treated with 10 million units/m², subcutaneously, three times weekly. Patients were treated for a minimum of three months. Doses were decreased to maintain a granulocyte count of more than 1,000, platelet count of more than 20,000 and SGOT less than 300 international units. Interferon treatment was discontinued in patients who had any severe adverse reactions.

Patients with high grade lymphoma were treated with 50 million units/m² per day given as a continuous intravenous infusion for five days. At institutions other than the UMCC, the total daily dose was sometimes administered as a single, 30 minute infusion. Cycles were repeated every three weeks, or sooner if there was complete recovery from any symptomatic or laboratory toxicities. Inital dose was decreased by individual investigators for patients with advanced age, lower performance status, or possible cardiovascular disease. At the University of Maryland Cancer Center, patients who had no dose limiting toxicities in the first cycle had dosage increased 25% in each subsequent cycle. Dosages were decreased in subsequent cycles if there were serious hematologic complications or hepatotoxicity.

Evaluation criteria and duration of treatment

Standard criteria were used to determine complete response, partial response, or stable disease. Patients were considered to have progressive disease if there was a 25% increase in tumor mass in any one site. In low grade lymphomas, patients received treatment for at least three months. Patients with stable disease or progressive disease had treatments stopped at this point and were observed. Patients with partial response received at least four months of treatment or at least three months of treatment following the documentation of maximum antitumor response. Patients with complete response received an additional two months of treatment. Patients with high grade lymphoma received at least two cycles of treatment beyond the time of maximum antilymphoma response. Patients with progressive disease at any time during treatment were removed from study and treated with other measures and are counted as treatment failures.

Results

Low grade histology lymphomas treated at the University of Maryland Cancer Center (Tables 1 & 2)

Thirteen patients were entered on study at the University of Maryland Cancer Center (Fig. 1). Ages ranged from 37 to 68 years (median 60). Twelve patients were evaluable. One patient developed a pulmonary embolus (probably from a deep venous thrombosis that was present before the beginning of treatment), received only two doses of interferon, and is considered inevaluable. Patients had advanced disease; 11 had stage IV disease at the time of treatment. The single patient with stage III disease is the only patient who did not have bone marrow involvement. One patient had liver involvement. The one patient with hairy cell leukemia had bone involvement. No patient had lymphoma in lung, skin or soft tissue. Eleven of the 13 had measurable lymph node involvement. Patients were heavily previously treated. Only two patients were previously untreated. Eleven patients had a median of two previous chemotherapy regimens; seven had received previous radiotherapy.

Five patients had IWF-A histology lymphomas (Fig. 2). This included one patient with relapsed Waldenstrom's macroglobulinemia with predominantly

Table 1. Low dose alpha-2 interferon: Low grade lymphomas at UMCC

Patients	13
Age (Median)	60
(Range)	37–68
Evaluable patients*	12
Stage IV	11
Previous treatment	
None	2
Chemotherapy (Median = 2)	11
Radiotherapy	7

*One patient inevaluable because of pulmonary embolus after 2 doses.

nodal and visceral infiltration as a manifestation of her disease. No responses were seen in this group of patients. (Fig. 2). Seven patients had nodular poorly differentiated lymphocytic lymphoma or nodular mixed lymphoma (IWF-B or C). Two patients achieved partial remission. One patient with nodular poorly differentiated lymphocytic lymphoma had previously untreated stage III A disease with only lymph node. His performance status was good (ECOG) [1]. Lymphoma had been first diagnosed two months prior to interferon treatment. The patient was treated with 10 million/m^2 per dose three times weekly. After three months of progressive improvement he had a 50% reduction in nodal mass. There was no further improvement in three months of subsequent treatment and interferon treatment was discontinued. Partial remission lasted for six months. The patient continued to be asymptomatic but had an increase in lymph node size. Although lymphoma has recurred, the patient had not received any subsequent treatment and continues to be well. During the treatment the patient had tolerable side effects except for a brief episode of mental confusion. It was felt that given the indolent course of his disease and the short period of continued response (three months), further treatment of his lymphoma with interferon was not advisable.

A patient with nodular mixed lymphoma achieved a partial response during interferon treatment. This 37-year-old man had relapsed stage IV B lymphoma with lymph node and marrow involvement. Previous treatment had included both radiotherapy and four different chemotherapy regimens, to all of which he was resistant. Because of previous treatment with total body irradiation, adequate doses of chemotherapy were complicated by prohibitive myelosuppression. The patient suffered significant symptomatic debility because of back pain due to paraspinal lymphadenopathy. Treatment was started with 10 million/m^2 per dose. No dosage reduction was required during treatment for either granulocytopenia or thrombocytopenia despite the previous poor tolerance to myelosuppressive chemotherapy. Following the initiation of treatment there was slow but

Table 2. Low dose alpha-2 interferon: Low grade lymphomas at UMCC

Classification (Rappaport)	No. (IWF)		Partial response	Duration (months)	Time to response	Off IFN
CLL, WDL, Waldenstrom's	A	5[a]	0	–	–	–
NPDL	B	5	1	6	3	9
NML	C	2[b]	1	11+	2	1
HCL		1	1	6+	2	–
		13[a, b]	3			

[a] One patient inevaluable (early pulmonary embolus).
[b] One patient inevaluable (wrong histology).

increasing response to treatment. By the end of two months there was a 50% reduction in tumor mass. The back pain from paraspinal adenopathy had decreased and the patient discontinued narcotic analgesics. His performance status steadily improved. After achieving partial remission, there continued to be further shrinkage of retroperitoneal lymph nodes in all groups. Bone marrow biopsy showed decrease in involvement with lymphoma, but a small focus of atypical lymphocytes compatible with lymphoma persisted. After 12 months of continuous treatment with interferon there had been no further nodal shrinkage for three months, and interferon treatment was discontinued. The patient remains in partial remission one month after interferon therapy was discontinued.

A single patient with hairy cell leukemia was also included in the study. He had advanced disease with extensive bone lesions. Involvement of vertebra and both femurs had led to pathological fracture which had been treated with radiotherapy. The patient had a transient improvement following splenectomy but then had pancytopenia with anemia that was entirely transfusion dependent. The patient had not responded to chemotherapy either with single alkylating agents or combination chemotherapy.

After two months of interferon treatment, the patient achieved a partial response. Hematocrit increased spontaneously without transfusion to greater than 40. White count and platelet count rose to normal levels. Prior to therapy, 45% of peripheral blood leukocytes were recognizable as typical hairy cells of leukemic reticuloendotheliosis and were stainable with tartrate resistant acid phosphatase. There was progressive decrease in the number of these cells. Currently, 7% of the white cell differential is either atypical lymphocytes or recognizable hairy cells. Successive bone marrow studies have shown steady improvement. Initially bone marrow had been inaspirable on numerous occasions. This corresponded to increased marrow fibrosis of moderate degree that was seen on reticulin stain. Bone marrow biopsy showed a round cell infiltrate, hypercellularity (3+/4+), and a decrease in normal hemopoietic elements. Successive bone marrow biopsies have shown that marrow fibrosis has steadily decreased and is now only mildly increased. Marrow can be readily aspirated. Bone marrow biopsy is normocellular. Although there are small, persistent foci of a round cell infiltrate, compatible with hairy cell leukemia, the areas of marrow that were replaced by hairy cell leukemia are no longer detectable. At this time, the patient continues to show improvement on each successive bone marrow biopsy and is tolerating continued interferon treatment which he has received now for more than eight months.

Symptomatic improvement has allowed the patient to return to work for the first time in years. For a brief period treatment was interrupted because of mild uticaria and macular, erythematous skin eruption that occurred after each interferon injection and lasted for 24 hours. The patient was retreated with a different interferon preparation that did not contain contaminating ampicillin, and he has had no subsequent recurrence of skin rash. Therapy was not interrupted for a transient increase in transaminase which resolved spontaneously on treatment.

Low grade lymphomas – collected multi center experience (Table 3)

Figure 3 shows the collected experience in the treatment of low grade lymphomas with alpha-2 at five cooperating centers. No responses were seen in lymphomas of histology IWF-A and none were treated with histology IWF-D. At the other four centers, responses were seen in an additional two patients with nodular mixed lymphoma and in an additional six patients with nodular poorly differentiated lymphocytic lymphoma. The overall response rate for all low grade non-Hodgkin's lymphomas is 45% with a median duration of seven months. In this study, responses were only seen in the nodular lymphomas.

Toxicity (Table 4)

The experience at the University of Maryland Cancer Center reflects the overall experience of the group, which has not yet been completely analyzed. All patients experienced a flu-like syndrome. Tolerance to these symptoms developed rapidly after the first two or three doses of interferon. In no patient were symptoms dose limiting nor did they lead to the cessation of treatment. Although bone marrow involvement was frequent in this group and patients had been heavily treated previously, myelosuppression was acceptable. Only one patient had dosage adjustment for neutropenia; two patients had doses lowered because of thrombocytopenia. This is in keeping with the experience in a previous phase I trial at the UMCC. Thrombocytopenia was only found to be dose limiting in interferon treatment in those patients who either had bone marrow involvement with malignancy or who had heavy previous treatment with chemotherapy and

Table 3. Alpha-2 interferon: Response in non-Hodgkin's lymphoma (low grade)

	NPDL	NML	NH	DWDL-CLL
Entered	17	4	0	7
Evaluable	14	3	–	3
Non-evaluable	1 skin rash	1 DX changed	–	1 infection
	1 fatigue			2 early death
	1 tete			1 pulm emb.
Time to response	2, 2, 3, 2, 2, 3	2, 2, 3	–	–
Duration	8, 7, 2, 6, 12+, 5+	8+, 2, 8+	–	–
PR	5	3	–	–
CR	1	–	–	–
NR	8	–	–	3

Table 4. Low dose alpha-2 interferon: Toxicity

Patients		13
Flu-like symptoms		13
Dose limiting		0
Neutropenia	– Grade 3 (<700/mm³)	2
	– Grade 4 (<500/mm³)	1
Platelets	– Grade 4(<25,000/mm³)	2
SGOT	– Grade 2 (80–300 IU)	5
	– Grade 3 (300–600 IU)	0
Mild confusion		2

radiotherapy. Hepatotoxicity was mild and did not require dosage adjustment. Two patients developed mild confusion. There were no other identifiable sources of the problem. Lumbar puncture and head CT scan were normal in both patients. Both patients had recovery while receiving interferon treatment.

High grade histology lymphomas treated at the University of Maryland Cancer Center (Tables 5 & 6)

Nine patients with high grade lymphoma were treated at the University of Maryland Cancer Center. The median age was 48 (range 16–73 years). Only one patient, with diffuse poorly differentiated lymphocytic lymphoma (IWF-E), stage IV-A, had received no previous treatment. Lymphoma was first diagnosed one month prior to treatment. Lymphoma involved lymph nodes and bone marrow and progressed following two cycles of treatment, despite increase of dose to 65 MU/m² by continuous intravenous infusion. The eight other patients had received one or two previous chemotherapeutic regimens; two patients had also received radiotherapy. Only three patients had previously achieved a complete response to treatment. Patients had advanced disease, with seven patients having stage IV disease. All had lymph node involvement. Six patients also had

Table 5. High dose alpha-2 interferon: High grade lymphomas at UMCC

Patients entered	9	Pleura	2
Age		Lung	1
(Median)	48	Bone	1
(Range)	16–73	Liver	1
Stage		Renal	1
III	2	Previous treatment	
IV	7	None	1
Involved sites		Chemotherapy (1 or 2)	8
Lymph node	9	Radiotherapy + CT	2
Marrow	6	Complete response	3

Table 6. High dose alpha-2 interferon: high grade lymphomas at UMC

Classification Rappaport	(IWF)	N	Evaluable[a]	Time to progression cycles
DPDL	E	3	2	2,3
DML	F	3	2	3,3
DHL	G	1	0	–
Imm. sarcoma	H	1	1	4
LL	I	1	1	3

[a] Inevaluable: One early death (GI bleed); Two patients with dyspnea and confusion.

involvement of bone marrow at the time of relapse. Three patients are not evaluable for treatment response. One patient developed acute upper gastrointestinal bleeding after the second day of treatment and aspirated gastric contents, suffering death from respiratory failure. Two patients developed dyspnea and confusion during the first day of high dose treatment and received no further treatment with interferon. In the six other patients, progressive disease developed following between two and four cycles of treatment. This occured even though most patients received escalated doses and even though treatment was given on schedule. In no patient was treatment delayed for more than four weeks following the previous cycle of chemotherapy. Despite this aggresive approach to treatment, there were no objective antitumor responses. A single patient with marrow lymphoblastic lymphoma had a transient decrease in bone marrow cellularity without a meaningful clinical improvement.

High grade lymphomas – collected multicenter experience (Table 7)

A total of 40 patients were entered at all participating centers. Only 29 of these patients are evaluable for treatment response. Three additional patients suffered early death from complications of rapidly progressive lymphoma. One patient had intolerable myelosuppression. Three patients became hypotensive from fluid loss, vasodilation, or rapid tachyarrhythmias. Response was observed in four patients (Fig. 7). A patient with diffuse poorly differentiated lymphocytic lymphoma is in continuing partial response at eight months. One patient with diffuse undifferentiated lymphoma with T-cell markers is in complete remission without evidence of disease at 18 months. Stage II disease, limited to abdominal lymph nodes, had relapsed following previous chemotherapy. She had treatment given both as continuous 24 hour infusion in five day cycles as well as courses of five daily 30 minute infusions.

Table 7. Alpha-2 interferon: response in non-Hodgkin's lymphoma (high grade)

	DPDL	DHL	DML	T-cell	Other
Entered	12	16	5	5	2 (immunoblastic; undiff.)
Evaluable	11	11	4	2	1
Non-evaluable	1 ALLERGIC	1 non-measurable 2 hypotension 1 hypertension 1 early death	1 hypotension	2 early death 1 inadequate marrow reserve (<1 cycle)	1 early death
Time to response	2	1,1	–	3	–
Duration	8^{+}	3,4	–	18^{+}	–
PR	1	2	–	–	–
CR	–	–	–	1	–
NR	10	9	4	2	2

The three patients who were inevaluable for response because of early toxicity were discussed previously. Additionally, one patient developed confusion several days following cessation of interferon treatment. This resolved slowly over several weeks and the patient was not retreated. Four patients developed granulocytopenia with less than 700 cells per cubic millimeter. In all these patients, recovery occurred rapidly following the completion of the five day course. No patient suffered a serious infection during granulocytopenia, although several minor infections occurred during periods off interferon treatment between cycles. Thrombocytopenia occurred in four patients, but did not require support with platelet transfusion. Myelosuppression was most severe in patients with marrow involvement and in whom previous chemotherapy had caused severe myelosuppression. Modest elevations of hepatic transaminases were frequent, but only two patients had elevations above 300 IU. In all patients there was prompt resolution of this abnormality following the completion of the five day cycle of treatment. A single patient developed mucositis with oral erythema and anal tenderness with some hematochezia. All patients had marked constitutional symptoms with high fever, myalgias and profound fatigue. Overall, the high rate and severity of complications was not justified by the low response rate in these patients.

Discussion

The non-Hodgkin's lymphomas are malignancies which are frequently responsive to a number of treatment modalities, including a number of chemotherapeutic agents. There is still an important need for new agents which are effective in lymphoma, especially for agents that have a unique mechanism of action or a range of toxicities different from those of standard chemotherapy. Preliminary experience suggested that the nodular lymphomas were particularly responsive to treatment with alpha interferon. This is confirmed in the experience both at the UMCC and in the larger group of five cooperating centers. The overall response rate in evaluable patients with low grade non-Hodgkin's lymphoma is 45%, with a median duration of response of seven months. Even if all patients who were entered on study are considered, the response rate remains 32%. This establishes a substantial rate of response to interferon in this group of patients, even though many had been previously treated. In low grade lymphomas, however, responses were limited to those patients with nodular lymphoma. No responses were seen in seven patients with chronic lymphocytic leukemia, diffuse well differentiated lymphoma or Waldenstrom's macroglobulinemia. Response was of particular clinical value in those patients who had lymphoma that was not responsive to treatment with conventional agents or in whom the toxicity of conventional treatment was prohibitive because of excessive myelosuppression. Overall, the lower doses of interferon administered in this study were well tolerated.

Rapid tolerance to the flu-like symptoms that accompany the initial treatment developed in all patients. Only one patient had treatment discontinued because of fatigue. Treatment with full dose was tolerated in some patients for as long as one year. This was important, because in several patients the maximum response to therapy occurred slowly and progressively over the course of many months. In one patient at the UMCC, response duration was short following discontinuation of therapy, and more prolonged treatment might have produced a more durable response.

These results confirm that alpha-2 interferon is an active agent in the treatment of nodular lymphoma. The mechanism of this antilymphoma action is not known. In other trials of alpha interferon given at these doses, no consistent immunostimulation has been detectable by *in vitro* measures of immunity [15]. It is also possible that interferon exerts a direct antiproliferative activity on lymphoma cells. Because interferon is such a potent modifier of the behavior of normal lymphocytes, it is possible that malignant lymphocytes are particularly responsive to its antiproliferative effects. It is not known whether the stage of B-cell differentiation which gives rise to nodular lymphomas is normally a cell which is particularly responsive to the action of interferon.

The overall response rate of high grade lymphomas to interferon is disappointingly small. Despite administration of maximally tolerated doses in an intensive schedule, there are few responses. Typically after only a few cycles of treatment there is disease progression without any evidence of transient response. However, there are individual patients that did derive substantial benefit from treatment. A patient with diffuse undifferentiated lymphoma with T-cell markers has had a complete remission lasting more than 18 months. This raises the possibility that high grade lymphomas are not a uniform group of diseases in their sensitivity to interferon treatment. It is possible that certain histologic subgroups or lymphomas with certain cell surface marker phenotypes will be more responsive to interferon treatment. A patient with diffuse poorly differentiated lymphocytic lymphoma has also had a partial remission, which has been durable for more than eight months. This is also a histology of lymphoma that is not of a uniform phenotype by cell surface markers. It is possible that further study will discover tests which are predictive of clinical response to interferon treatment.

The toxicity of high dose treatment with interferon is substantial, whether given either by continuous infusion or by daily 30 minute infusions. It is certain that drug toxicity contributed to the large number of patients that were inevaluable in this group of patients. However, relapsed high grade lymphoma is frequently a rapidly progressive disease. This also contributed to the large number of patients who were not completely evaluable for response. In particular, high fever, cardiovascular problems and neurological toxicity with confusion were the most serious problems from high dose treatment. Although myelosuppression was frequent and sometimes required dose reductions, only one patient had treatment discontinued altogether because of inadequate marrow reserve. In general, there is rapid recovery from myelosuppression. Mild to moderate hepatotoxicity as evidenced by transaminase elevations also occurred frequently but was not dose limiting and was rapidly reversible.

In this multicenter experience with alpha-2 interferon in the United States, we conclude that treatment was well tolerated in patients who received low dose by the subcutaneous route, but less well tolerated by patients receiving high dose intravenous treatment. Most toxicity was reversible with cessation of treatment. Despite toxicity, low dose treatment can be given for prolonged periods of time. The response rate in low grade non-Hodgkin's lymphoma is 45% with a median duration of seven months. Responses were seen only in patients with nodular lymphomas. The overall response rate in patients with high grade non-Hodgkin's lymphoma is 13%. The low response rate is partially accounted for by the intense treatment which patients had generally received previously and to which they were refractory. Although the overall response rate is low in high grade non-Hodgkin's lymphoma, further study is necessary to determine if certain histologic subtypes or other prognostic features predict a higher response to interferon therapy.

References

1. Portlock CS: Deferral of initial therapy for advanced indolent lymphomas. Cancer Treatment Rep 66:417-419, 1982.
2. Streuli RA, Ultmann JE: Non-Hodgkin's lymphomas: Historical perspective and future prospects. Semin Oncol 7:223-233, 1980.

3. Schein PS, Chabner BA, Canellos GP, *et al:* Potential for prolonged disease-free survival following combination chemotherapy of non-Hodgkin's lymphoma. Blood 43:181-189, 1978.

4. Anderson T, Bender RA, Fisher RI, *et al:* Combination chemotherapy in non-Hodgkin's lymphomas: Result of long-term followup. Cancer Treat Rep 61:1057–1066, 1977.

5. Diggs CH, Wiernik PH, Ostrow SS: Nodular lymphoma: Prolongation of survival by complete remission. Cancer Clin Trials 4:107-114, 1981.

6. Ezdinli EZ, Costello W, Glick JH: Nodular non-Hodgkin's lymphomas: Effect of histologic pattern and response on survival. Proc Amer Assoc Cancer Res and ASCO 22:516, 1981.

7. Glick JH, Barnes JM, Ezdinli EZ, Berard CW, Orlow EL, Bennett JM: Nodular mixed lymphoma: Results of a randomized trial failing to confirm prolonged disease-free survival with COPP chemotherapy. Blood 58: 920-925, 1981.

8. Rosenberg SA, Berard CW, Brown BW Jr, *et al:* National Cancer Institute sponsored study of classifications of non-Hodgkin's lymphomas. Cancer 49:2112–2135, 1982.

9. Merigan TC, Sikora K, Breeden JH, Levy R, Rosenberg SA: Preliminary observations on the effect of human leukocyte interferon in non-Hodgkin's lymphoma. N Engl J Med 299:1449-1453, 1978.

10. Gutterman IU, Blumenshein GR, Alexanian R, Yap HY, Buzdar AU, Cabanillas F, Hortobagyi GN, Hersh EM, Rasmussen SL, Harmon M, Kramer M, Pestka S: Leukocyte interferon-induced tumor regression in human metastatic breast cancer, multiple myeloma, and malignant lymphoma. Ann Intern Med 93:399-406, 1980.

11. Leavitt RD, Duffey PL, Wiernik PH, Fein S, Sherwin S, Scogna D, Oldham R: A phase I trial of twice daily recombinant human leukocyte A interferon (IFL-rA) in cancer patients. Proc Am Soc Clin Oncol 1:41, 1982.

12. Sherwin S, Knost J, Fein S, Abrams P, Foon K, Ochs J, Schoenberger C, Oldham R: A multiple dose phase I trial of recombinant leukocyte A interferon using a 3 × weekly schedule. Proc Am Soc Clin Oncol 1:35, 1982.

13. Quesada Jr, Gutterman JU, Fein S: A phase I study of recombinant DNA produced leukocyte interferon by an intermittent schedule. Proc Am Soc Clin Oncol 1:36, 1982.

14. Horning SJ, Levine JF, Miller RA, Merigan TC: Clinical immunologic effects of recombinant leukocyte A interferon in eight patients with advanced cancer. Second Annual International Congress for Interferon Research, Oct. 21–23, San Francisco, Calif., 1981.

15. Maluish AE, Conlon J, Ortaldo JR, Sherwin SA, Leavitt RD, Fein S, Wiernik PH, Oldham RK, Herberman RB: Depression of natural killer cytotoxicity after *in vivo* administration of recombinant leukocyte interferon. J Immunol 131:503-507, 1983.

8. Use in patients with resistant and relapsing Multiple Myeloma. A Phase II Study

J. COSTANZI, M.R. COOPER, J.H. SCARFFE, H. OZER, R.B. POLLARD, R.W. FERRARESI and R.J. SPIEGEL

Abstract

The use of phenylalanine mustard or cyclophosphamide alone and in various combination chemotherapy programs has improved the response rate and disease-free survival in multiple myeloma. However, once those patients have become refractory or have relapsed on that therapy, subsequent salvage treatment has been very disappointing. Between 1979 and 1982 a number of preliminary studies were reported using human leukocyte interferon (Cantell) in patients with refractory or relapsing myeloma. The total number of patients reported in those studies was 25. Five of these patients had a partial response. Therefore, the present study utilizing Schering human alpha-2 interferon, was undertaken in a multi-institutional program. Thirty-eight fully evaluable patients were treated with three different alpha-2 interferon schedules. Seven of these patients had a response with one a complete remission. Of the seven responders, two were from 19 refractory patients and five from 19 relapsing patients. The complete response continues in maintained remission at 72+ weeks with the other responders lasting from 12 to 58+ weeks. In most of these patients an improvement in performance status and bone pain was noted.

Almost all patients experienced some form of fatigue and flu-like symptoms. Two-third of the patients noted anorexia and 25 to 33% of the patients experienced some degree of confusion, somnolence, dry mouth, depression and hypotension. Leukopenia was seen in half of the patients and one-third of the patients experienced thrombocytopenia and anemia. A very small number of patients had transient abnormalities in various chemistries including LDH, SGOT, SGPT, alkaline phosphatase and creatinine.

Schering human alpha-2 interferon appears effective in resistant and relapsing patients with multiple myeloma. These studies are being continued and the combination of chemotherapy plus interferon is being considered for previously untreated patients.

Introduction

The introduction of alkylating agents in the treatment of multiple myeloma clearly improved the response rate [1]. These alkylating agents also increased the median survival time from diagnosis [2]. Unfortunately this median survival of 24 to 33 months has plateaued even with the use of four or five drug induction regimens [2, 3].

In patients who have relapsed or have become refractory to these treatments, subsequent salvage therapy have been largely unsuccessful [4–10]. A number of new phase II chemotherapeutic agents have been utilized in the treatment of myeloma in patients who have become resistant or have relapsed. Some of these agents include DHAD, Bisantrene, m-AMSA and Aclacinomycin. These agents have produced very minimal to no responses. It is clear that newer active compounds are needed in this disease.

With the availability of interferon, a smal number of studies were reported between 1979 and 1982 using primarily human leukocyte interferon (Cantell) [11–14]. In these reports there were a total of 25 multiple myeloma patients who had relapsed or were unresponsive to primary therapy. Of these 25 patients, five were reported to have a partial response, thus confirming the activity of interferon in the treatment of some patients with multiple myeloma. While the results of those studies utilizing natural interferon must be regarded as preliminary, this form of therapy clearly influenced the level of abnormal serum proteins and modified the course of the disease in those patients.

This study reports the results of a multi-institutional phase II clinical trial utilizing recombinant alpha-2 interferon in 49 patients with relapsing or resistant multiple myeloma.

Materials and methods

Patients entering this study were diagnosed according to the criteria of the myeloma study task force and staged according to the criteria of Durie and Salmon [15, 16]. Only patients refractory to prior therapy or relapsing after an initial response to primary therapy were entered. Patients were required to have a life expectancy of at least 4 months and an ECOG performance status of 0, 1, 2 or 3. No concomitant therapy was allowed, including radiation therapy. The demographic characteristics of patients entered are listed in Table 1.

Interferon, used in this study, is a highly purified human alpha-2 interferon produced by recombinant DNA-techniques in *E. coli* [17]. alpha-2 interferon (Schering Sch 30500) was administered in three different dose schedules (Table 2). Four centers used a similar schedule of daily intravenous induction followed by subcutaneous 3 ×/week maintenance therapy. The fifth center (H.S.) used subcutaneous alpha-2 interferon from the beginning of therapy. As each schedule

Table 1. Phase II myeloma trials

	Patient characteristics
Entered	49
Evaluable	38
Age	63 (33–80)
Sex	29 F, 20 M
PS	0=11, 1=16, 2=17, 3=5
M protein	IgG 28
	IgA 12
	light chain 7
	non-secretor 2
Light chain	37 Kappa, 11 Lambda, 1 NA
Prior response	refractory 26
	relapsing 23 (16 on Rx, 7 off Rx)
Prior Rx	M-P 7
	M-P-C 10
	mult. drugs 32

had similar toxicity and produced response rates not statistically significantly different from each other, results of all studies are combined in this report.

Pre-treatment and post-treatment serum specimens were assayed by means of radioimmunoassay and bioassay for interferon neutralizing activity. The screen for interferon neutralizing factors in human sera was done by a competitive assay using a modification of the Celltech Interferon Immunoradiometric Assay and Sch 30500. The diluted serum samples were allowed to react with a fixed amount of interferon, then ^{125}I-anti-alpha interferon monoclonal antibody was added, followed by a polystyrene bead coated with polyclonal anti-alpha interferon antibody. After 3–4 hours at ambient temperature, the mixtures are incubated at 4–6°C overnight. Any interferon which has not been "neutralized" by the serum will react with the labelled monoclonal antibody and link it to the bead. The radioactivity bound to the bead is compared to that of a standard curve prepared at the same time in the presence of pooled, non-immune human sera. A 50% or greater reduction in detectable alpha-2 interferon, as compared to the standard, is considered positive for neutralizing factor. This assay can detect 50 units/ml or greater neutralizing activity.

Table 2. Phase II MYELOMA TRIALS

	Enrolled	Evaluable
3–100 × 10^6 IU/m²/d I.V. × 2 wks	23	18
10 × 10^6 IU/m² S.C. TIW		
30–50 × 10^6 IU/m²/d I.V., 5 on/9 off × 4	12	7
10 × 10^6 IU/m² S.C. TIW		
2 × 10^6/m²/d S.C. TIW	14	13
	49	38

Response criteria utilized were those recommended by the Chronic Myeloma Task Force Study Group [15]. A complete response (CR) was defined as the disappearance of serum paraprotein measured by at least two serum protein electrophoretic determination four weeks apart and a qualitative immunoelectrophoresis. If present, a decrease in urinary light chain protein (Bence-Jones proteins) to 0.1 g/24 h was required on two determinations, as well as the disappearance of any soft tissue masses. Additional criteria included a return of hematological parameters to normal values. A partial response (PR) was defined as a decrease in the serum paraprotein to 50% or more below the pre-treatment level as measured by at least two serum protein electrophoretic determinations four weeks apart. If urinary light chains were present, the decrease had to be 50% or more below pre-treatment levels based on at least two determinations. Bone marrow determinations, although performed, were not required to determine a partial remission. Changes in the serum monoclonal protein or urine monoclonal protein greater than 25% but less than 50% if the pre-study determinations were categorized as minor responses.

Actual survival curves were compared utilizing generalized Wilcoxan (Breslow) and Savage (Mantel-Cox) statistics [18, 19].

Results

Forty-nine eligible patients were entered into study of whom 38 were evaluable for efficacy analysis. Patients were considered invalid for response assessment if they had received less than one month of treatment. This occurred in nine patients for the following reasons: One patient was not eligible because he was irradiated less than 28 days before interferon treatment; six patients were removed from study (one refused further treatment, two had intercurrent illnesses not related to interferon, and three had adverse experiences possibly related to interferon – severe fatigue, paralytic ileus, and congestive heart failure); four patients died (two with disease progression, one with sepsis, and one with probable pneumonia and respiratory arrest). These patients will be evaluated for toxicity.

Demographics of the patient population are presented in Table 1. Two-thirds of the patients entered had been treated previously with multiple drug combinations including agents such as adriamycin, vincristine and nitrosoureas in addition to melphalan, cytoxan, and prednisone. At entry, 26/49 patients were refractory to all prior chemotherapy, whereas 23 were relapsing after having previously responded to chemotherapy. Of the 38 evaluable patients there were a total of seven responders (18%). There was one patient with a complete response and six partial responders (Tables 3 & 4). Variable response rates among patients from different prognostic sub-groups were noted. Among refractory patients who had never responded to prior therapy, there were 2/19 (10.5%) responses, whereas, among patients who had previously responded, there were 5/19 responses (26%). Three of six patients who had relapsed while off chemotherapy responded to interferon treatment. The amount of prior treatment also profoundly affected the response rate to interferon. Two of five patients who previously received alkylating agent plus prednisone responded to interferon, whereas only three of 25 patients who had failed multiple alkylating agent therapy responded to interferon.

Three of the seven responders continue to respond for greater than one year on continued maintenance therapy. One patient had a partial response for 40 weeks and then converted to a complete response with disappearance of abnormal M-protein and radiographic confirmation of healing lytic bone lesions. This CR now continues at 72+ weeks. In addition to the seven patients who had responses by conventional criteria there were an additional 13 patients who had at least a 25% decrease in their abnormal paraprotein documented on at least one follow-up visit (minor response). Additionally, a number of patients who did not meet response criteria for improvement in abnormal protein did have subjective improvement in bone pain during the course of interferon treatment (Table 5). Of 29 patients who entered the study with documented bone pain, 18 improved and 10 remained unchanged during the course of treatment. Only one patient had worsening of bone pain during interferon treatment.

Survival curves reveal a median survival for non-responders of 6.9 months versus 11.3+ months for responders and 15.4 months for patients who meet minor response criteria. These are statistically significant differences ($p<.05$) for Responders and Minor Responders vs. Non-responders. Despite the known limitations of this type of analysis, this finding suggests that the attainment of a response might give survival benefit.

Interferon therapy was well tolerated in the schedule used with only four patients discontinuing therapy due to adverse effects. Hematologic and non-hematologic toxicity was more severe during the induction phase than during the maintenance phase when patients had doses titrated to their maximum tolerated dose. In almost all cases it was possible to titrate individual patients' doses to a tolerable level. Non-hematologic toxicities are presented in Table 6. The most

Table 3. Phase II multiple myeloma trials

	Results	1,2
Refractory pts.	2/19	11%
Relapsing pts. (on Rx 2/13, off Rx 3/6)	5/19	26%
Minimal response	13/38	34%
Prior Rx: single agent	2/5	40%
M+C+P	2/8	25%
mult. agents	3/25	12%

1. Strict response criteria: > 50% decrease × 4 wks.
2. Follow-up: 3/7 relapses, others remain in remission 52+, 58+, 72+ WKS.

Table 4. Profile of responders

No.	Prior Rx	Stage	Response	Duration of response (weeks)	Best change in performance	Best change in pain	Type of protein
Costanzi							
PT. 4	Melphalan/prednisone	I	PR	58+	no change	no pain*	IGG
PT. 6	multiple drug	III	CR	72+	no change	improved (mild to none)	IGG
PT 14	multiple drug	III	PR	21	improved (2 to 1)	improved (mod. to none)	IGG
Cooper							
PT. 14	multiple drug	II	PR	52+	no change	improved (mod. to mild)	IGA
PT. 5A	melphalan/prednisone	II	PR	15	improved (3 to 1)	improved (mod. to mild)	IGA
Scarffe							
PT. 5	melphalan/prednisone & cytoxan/prednisone	III	PR	12	no change	no change	LTC(K)
PT. 6	melphalan/prednisone & cytoxan/prednisone	II	PR	16	no change	improved (mild to none)	IGG

* at baseline

commonly occurring side effect was a complex of constitutional symptoms characterized as "flu-like" (fever, malaise, anorexia). Some aspect of this flu-like syndrome occurred in over 90% of patients. During induction, 46% of patients reported these symptoms to be moderate to severe, but only 13% had these persistently during maintenance. Other significant non-hematologic toxicities included confusion and somnolence. These were completely reversible upon temporary cessation of interferon therapy. Similarly, elevated hepatic transaminases were observed in four patients during IV induction but resolved promptly upon discontinuation of interferon. These patients received lower doses of interferon during maintenance therapy without subsequent elevation of liver enzymes.

Table 5. Bone pain improvement

Bone pain	CR or PR	NC	PD	Total
Improved	5	3	10	18
Stable	1	4	5	10
Worse	0	1	0	1
	6	8	15	29

CR	– Complete Response
PR	– Partial Response
NC	– No Change/Minor Response
PD	– Progressive Disease

Table 6. Non-hematologic toxicity (% patients)

	Dose adjustment		Maintenance	
	All	Grades 3&4	All	Grades 3&4
Flu-like symptoms	97.7	45.5	73.3	13.3
Fatigue	84.1	27.3	66.7	16.7
Confusion	25.0	6.8	6.7	6.7
Anorexia	65.9	18.2	46.7	10.0
Diarrhea	38.6	6.8	16.7	0.0
Somnolence	40.9	9.1	30.0	13.3
Dry mouth	36.4	2.3	13.3	0.0
Depression	13.6	4.5	16.7	3.3
Hypotension	9.1	2.3	0.0	0.0

Table 7. Hematologic toxicity: Patients grade 0, 1 or 2; change to grade 3 or 4

	Dose adjustment		Maintenance	
		%		%
Hgb	11/37	29.7	9/27	33.3
WBC	22/39	56.4	8/25	32.0
Platelets	11/36	30.6	5/27	18.5
LDH	1/35	2.9	0/24	0.0
SGOT	3/42	7.1	0/30	0.0
SGPT	1/25	4.0	0/21	0.0
ALK PHOS	1/42	2.4	0/30	0.0
Creatinine	3/42	7.1	3/30	10.0
Bun	0/41	0.0	0/29	0.0

Hematologic and hepatic toxicity was strongly related to baseline hematologic parameters (Table 7). In patients who began with WBC >2000, 54% had nadirs <2000 during maintenance and 32% of patients had nadirs that required dose adjustment. Similarly, among patients with baseline platelet counts >50,000, 31% had nadirs <50,000 after interferon therapy. There was no evidence of cumulative hematologic toxicity.

No patients were documented to have developed serum neutralizing factors to interferon during the course of treatment.

Discussion

Several different approaches have been taken in the management of patients with relapsing or refractory myeloma. Prognostic factors in this group include reponse to prior therapy and amount of prior therapy. In truly refractory patients, no single drugs have demonstrated a >10% response rate. Even in the most favorable relapsing group, second-line therapies only give responses in the 25–35% range and even these results have not been consistently reproduced in confirmatory studies [2, 7]. In 1972, Bersagel *et al.* reported that high-dose intermittent cyclophosphamide was effective in patients who had demonstrated resistance to L-PAM [5]. More recent studies indicate cross-resistance between melphalan and cyclophosphamide and suggest that single alkylating agents cannot be recommended as second-line treatment for patients who are refractory to a prior alkylating agent [4, 6]. Other salvage regimens for relapsing or refractory myeloma patients have included non-alkylating agents and the combination of multiple drugs.

As single agents, non-alkylating drugs have been disappointing. In a study by Bennet *et al*, eight resistant patients received adriamycin and 19 received bleomycin; one partial response was seen with each agent, and the duration of both responses was less than 4 months [7]. Two recent Cancer and Leukemia Group B (CALGB) studies tested M-AMSA (methanesulfon-M anisidide) and AZQ (Azridinyl-Benzoquinone) in alkylating agent resistant myeloma. Of 68 evaluable patients who received M-AMSA, only four patients had objective responses. Median survival was only 2.9 months. AZQ was similarly disappointing: objective responses were not seen in any of the 32 patients evaluated and median survival was 3.6 months [20].

Hexamethylmelamine was another new drug of interest in the treatment of myeloma refractory to alkylating agents because of early encouraging results in lymphoma. Cohen *et al.* [8] reported that of 65 evaluable patients treated with hexamethylmelamine and prednisone, 35% experienced some response. Responders had a median survival of 19 months compared to non-responder's 6 months. Although the investigators concluded that hexamethylmelamine had some anti-tumor effect in myeloma, the drug's toxicity was significant, thereby limiting its general usefulness in the treatment of myeloma.

Multiple drug regimens have also been largely unrewarding. Presant and Klahr used a combination of adriamycin, BCNU, cyclophosphamide, and prednisone in 14 patients with myeloma resistant to L-PAM and prednisone [9]. Five of 14 patients had objective responses and those who responded had a median survival of 12.9 months while non-responders had a median survival of 3.4 months. CALGB conducted a trial in 89 patients resistant to L-PAM [21]. Patients were randomized to receive cyclophosphamide and prednisone or cyclophosphamide, BCNU and prednisone. Only 17% of patients receiving the two alkylators and 7% receiving the single alkylator had objective responses. Although responders had a median survival of 31 months vs 9.4 months in non-responders, the study concluded that due to toxicity, the addition of BCNU to cyclophosphamide could not be recommended in the face of minimal clinical gain. The Southwest Oncology Group used vincristine, BCNU, Doxorubicin and prednisone for salvage of patients with relapsing or refractory myeloma; approximately 25% of 151 patients had an objective response [22]. Patients who had previously responded to alkylating agent therapy had a 30% response rate to the combination program whereas those who had not previously responded to alkylating agents had only a

7% chance of response. The median survival for non-responders was 33 weeks compared to 78 weeks for responders.

Prior results with interferon have been limited but encouraging. Mellstedt *et al.* administered human leukocyte interferon to four previously untreated patients with multiple myeloma. All patients showed a decrease in the percentage of bone marrow plasma cells as well as a decrease in the level of abnormal proteins both in serum and urine [14]. Gutterman *et al* treated 10 myeloma patients with natural interferon; three responded, three improved, and four failed to respond [11]. The responders had decreases in abnormal proteins which lasted up to 63 weeks after therapy was discontinued and decreases in the percentage of plasma cells to 15% or less. Other small series of interferon treatments in myeloma patients have recently been reviewed [12]. Scandinavian investigators have reported a randomized trial comparing interferon alone with intermittent high dose melphalan and prednisone as first-line therapy [12]. Six of 21 evaluable patients in the chemotherapy group and 4/22 in the interferon group were classified as responders. The actuarial survival curves showed no statistically significant difference.

This multi-institutional trial utilizing recombinant alpha-2 interferon confirms the effectiveness of interferon in the management of patients with relapsing or refractory multiple myeloma. Although two-thirds of the patient population had received extensive prior treatment, 7/38 patients responded.

Three of the seven responders have had a survival time of greater than one year with marked improvement in performance status. One patient has achieved a durable and ongoing complete remission, which is rarely seen with either radiation therapy or chemotherapy. If the patients are analyzed according to prior treatment, one finds a 50% response rate for patients who had previously received only melphalan and prednisone, compared to 25% for those who had received multiple alkylators and 12% for patients who had received multiple alkylators plus other chemotherapeutic agents.

The interferon was generally well tolerated and only four patients left the trial due to non-compliance. Fever, lethargy and other flu-like syndromes were frequently noted, but were rarely dose limiting. Interferon was well tolerated during the long periods of treatment in the maintenance phase.

Although leukopenia and thrombocytopenia were noted in this patient population, it was not as severe as that seen with other chemotherapeutic agents and rarely was a dose limiting factor in treatment. The effectiveness of this recombinant alpha-2 interferon in a population of extensively pre-treated resistant and relapsing patients suggests that additional trials are warranted to study the effects of alpha-2 interferon in previously untreated patients either as a single agent or in combination with standard alkylating agent therapy.

References

1. Bergsagel DE, Sprague CC, Austin C: Evaluation of new chemotherapeutic agents in the treatment of multiple myeloma, IV. (L-phenylalanine mustard NSC-8806). Cancer Chemother Rep 21: 87-99, 1962.
2. Durie BGM, Salmon SE: The current status and future prospects of treatment for multiple myeloma. Clin Haematol 11:181-210, 1982.
3. Bergsagel D: Progress in the treatment of plasma cell myeloma? J Clin Onco 1:510-512, 1983.
4. Blade J, Feliue, Rozman C: Cross-resistance to alkylating agents in multiple myeloma. Cancer 52(5):786-789, 1983.
5. Bergsagel DE, Cowan DH, Hasselback R: Plasma cell myeloma: Response of melphalan-resistant patients to high-dose intermittent cyclophosphamide. C.M.A. Journal 101;851-855.
6. White D, Bergsagel D, Rapp EF: Failure of cyclophosphamide to produce response in melphalan-resistant multiple myeloma. Blood 58 (Suppl.):169a, 1981.
7. Bennett JM, Silver R, Ezdinli E: Phase II study of adriamycin and bleomycin in patients with multiple myeloma. Cancer Treat Rep 62:1367-1369, 1978.
8. Cohen JH, Bartolucci AA: Hexamethylmelamine and prednisone in the treatment of refractory multiple myeloma. Amer J Clin Oncol 5:21-27, 1972.
9. Presant CA, Klahr C: Adriamycin, 1-3-bis (2-chloroethyl)-1-nitrosourea (BCNU, NSC # 409962) cyclophosphamide plus prednisone (ABC-P) in melphalan-resistant multiple myeloma. Cancer 42:1222-1227, 1978.
10. Lake-Lewin D, Myers J, Lee BJ: Phase II trial of pyrazofurin in patients with multiple myeloma refractory to standard cytotoxic therapy. Cancer Treat Rep 63:1403-1404, 1979.
11. Gutterman JU, Blumenschein GR, Alexanian R: Leukocyte interferon-induced tumor regression in human metastatic breast cancer, multiple myeloma, and malignant lymphoma. Ann Intern Med 93:399-406, 1980.
12. Mellstedt H, Aahre, A, Bjorkholm M: Interferon therapy of patients with myeloma. In Immunotherapy of Human Cancer, Terry/Rosenberg (eds.) Elsevier North Holland, 1980, pp. 387-391.
13. Alexanian R, Gutterman J, Levy H: Interferon treatment for multiple myeloma. Clin Haematol 11:211, 1982.
14. Mellstedt H, Bjorkholm M, Johansson B: Interferon therapy in myelomatosis. Lancet I:245-248, 1979.
15. Chronic Leukemia-Myeloma Task Force, National Cancer Institute. Proposed guidelines for protocol studies II. Plasma cell myeloma. Cancer Chemother. Rep 4:145-158, 1973.
16. Durie BGM, Salmon SE: A clinical staging system for multiple myeloma. Correlation of measured myeloma cell mass with presenting clinical features, response to treatment and survival. Cancer 36:842-852, 1975.

17. Struli M, Nagata S, Weissman C: At least three human type alpha interferon: Structure of alpha 2. Science 209-1343, 1980.
18. Breslow N: A generalized Kurskal-Wallis test for comparing K samples subject to unequal patterns of censorship. Biometrika 57:579-594, 1970.
19. Mantel N: Evaluation of survival data and two new rank order statistics arising in its consideration. Cancer Chemother Rep 50:163-170, 1966.
20. Vinciguerra V, Anderson K, McIntyre OR: Azridinyl-BGNZ (AZQ) for resistant multiple myeloma. In press.
21. Kyle RA, Gailani S, Seligman BR: Multiple myeloma resistant to melphalan: Treatment with cyclophosphamide, prednisone and BCNU. Cancer Treat Rep 63:1265-1269, 1979.
22. Bonnet J, Alexanian R, Salmon S: Vincristine, BCNU, adriamycin, prednisone (VBAP), combination in the treatment of relapsing or resistant multiple myeloma. A Southwest Oncology Group Study. Cancer Treat Rep 66:1267-1271, 1982.

9. Use in Hairy Cell Leukemia. An Update*

H . M . G O L O M B , and M . J . R A T A I N

Abstract

Hairy Cell Leukemia (HCL) is a chronic lymphoproliferative disease which usually responds to splenectomy in the majority of patients. However, one-third of splenectomized patients subsequently develop increasing bone marrow involvement and signs of marrow underproduction. Since October, 1983, we have identified 16 patients with progressive HCL who have qualified for a trial of subcutaneous alpha-2 interferon. Of the 16 patients, the median age was 47 years, there were 12 males and 4 females, and 15 of 16 had had a previous splenectomy. In addition, 10 of 16 had been previously treated with chlorambucil. At the time of initiation of IFN, 14 of 16 were anemic (Hb<12), 10 of 16 were thrombocytopenic (plts<100,000) and all 16 were neutropenic (Neutrophils<1,000). Four patients had the leukemic phase (wbc>10,000 c 50% or more hairy cells). Patients 1–4 and 6 received an initial dose of 10 million u/m^2, and the remainder of the patients received 2 million u/m^2. Patients 1–4 subsequently had a dose reduction to 2–4 million u/m^2. Patient 6 died during the first week of therapy due to an intracerebral hemorrhage; she was refractory to platelets when first referred.

Nine patients are eligible for consideration at this point (greater than 8 weeks since initial therapy); patient 6 is excluded and thus 8 are evaluable. Two patients had a partial response, 5 patients had a minor response, and 1 patient had no objective response. Resolution of significant neutropenia was seen in 6 to 8 patients. Objective assessment of the bone marrow showed a marked decrease in the cellularity in 7 of the 8 evaluable cases with a concomitant decrease in hairy cell involvement. Toxicity was mild with fever in all 8 patients, fatigue in 7, and myalgias in 5. An influenza-like syndrome was seen in 4 patients.

We conclude that alpha-2 interferon is effective in HCL; the percentage of responding patients needs to be determined as does the length of treatment necessary to assure a response. The duration of a response remains to be defined.

* Supported in part by Harry Greenberg Foundation, Bellman Research Fund and Schering Corp.

Introduction

Hairy cell leukemia (HCL) is a chronic lymphoproliferative disease which requires accurate diagnosis based on a biopsy of the bone marrow [1]. The diagnosis can be suspected on the basis of the clinical presentation of splenomegaly without adenopathy, and pancytopenia as well as the morphologic characteristics of circulating "hairy" cells, but bone marrow biopsy tissue must be obtained. Once the diagnosis is confirmed, the pace of the disease should be established prior to initiating therapy. The accepted first-line treatment for patients requiring therapy is splenectomy [2].

Subsequently, one-third of post-splenectomy patients will develop progressive disease characterized by either a leukemic phase with associated cytopenias or progressive pancytopenia in association with increasing replacement of the bone marrow by hairy cells [3]. Thus, the hairy cells have to be eradicated from the bone marrow in order to reverse the underproduction problem. From 1975 through 1984, we utilized the alkylating agent chlorambucil in low daily dosage (4 mg) to slowly remove the hairy cells from the bone marrow [4]. This approach was successful in reversing the anemia and thrombocytopenia in the majority of patients, but persistent granulocytopenia left the patients susceptable to serious, systemic infections which could be life-threatening. In 1984, Quesada *et al* reported on 7 HCL patients treated with purified leukocyte interferon [5]. Although several of the patients had relatively normal blood counts initially and would not have required chlorambucil therapy, two gratifying results were seen. There was a dramatic increase in the absolute granulocyte count over several months and 3 of the patients were reported to have complete eradication of hairy cells from their bone marrow. These unexpected findings led to the initiation of further trials utilizing interferon in the treatment of HCL. The development of recombinant interferon (Schering Corp.) permitted several centers to initiate clinical trials beginning in late 1983.

Methods

At the University of Chicago between October 1983 and April 1984, we have entered 16 patients with progressive hairy cell leukemia into an alpha-interferon trial. Alpha 2 interferon was obtained from the Schering Corporation (Kenilworth, N.J.) as the lyophilized powder (10×10^6 and 50×10^6 international units per vial), reconstituted with sterile water, and administered subcutaneously. Informed consent for participation in the study was obtained from patients prior to treatment. Our criteria for inclusion included: a pathologically confirmed diagnosis of HCL on the basis of a bone core biopsy performed within one month of entry, progressive cytopenia(s) following splenectomy (except one patient who refused splenectomy for severe thrombocytopenia), normal hepatic and renal function, no previous therapy for one month, and no prior or concomitant malignant disorder (excluding basal cell carcinoma). Five of the first 6 patients were started on IFN at a dose of $10 \times 10^6 U/m^2$ three times per week; the remaining patients were started at $2 \times 10^6 U/m^2$ three times per week. Initially, the first three injections were administered under direct supervision, with monitoring for 6 hours. Subsequently, two injections were supervised with monitoring for 1 hour. Patients were premedicated with acetaminophen, 650 mg.

Complete blood counts including differential obtained weekly. Bone marrow biopsies were performed monthly, with assessment of cellularity and percentage of hairy cells. The hairy cell index (HCI), defined as

$$(\frac{\% \text{ cellularity} \times \% \text{ hairy cells}}{10,000})$$ was determined [3].

Criteria for response were similar to those established by Quesada *et al.* [5] and defined as follows:

Complete Response (CR) – a) an absence of hairy cells in the bone marrow core biopsy *and* b) improvement in the peripheral blood counts to hemoglobin > 12g/dl, platelets > 100,000 cells/cu mm, and neutrophils > 1500 cells/cu mm.

Partial Response (PR) – a) an absence of hairy cells in the peripheral blood *and* b) improvement in the peripheral blood counts as indicated above.

Minor Response (MR) – a) improvement in hemoglobin to more than 10g/dl (without transfusions) *or* b) improvement in platelets to more than 100,000 cells/cu mm *or* c) improvement in neutrophils to more than 1000 cells/cu mm *or* d) decrease in hairy cells (*if* initially leukemic) to less than 5% of peripheral white cells.

Patient characteristics

The 16 patients ranged in age from 33 to 71 years with a median of 47 years. There were 12 men and 4 women. Fifteen had had a previous splenectomy; one patient refused initial splenectomy therapy for his severe thrombocytopenia. Of the 15 patients who had undergone previous splenectomy, responses as judged by the above criteria were: 0 complete responses, 1 partial response, 13 marginal responses, and 1 no response. The median time since splenectomy to progression was 27 months with a range of 4 to 163 months. Ten patients (63%) had been previously treated with chlorambucil; 5 demonstrated a marginal response and 5 had no response. At the time of entry on the IFN study, 14 had a hemoglobin < 12 g/dl; 6 patients had a transfusion requirement. Ten patients had a platelet count less than 100,000/mm³; 8 of these were less than 50,000/mm³ and 6 patients required platelet transfusions. All 16 patients were neutropenic (granulocytes < 1000/mm³) and 12 had a granulocyte count < 500/mm³. Four patients had a white blood count (WBC) > 10,000/mm³ with greater than 50% hairy cells.

Preliminary results

Nine of the 16 patients were eligible for evaluation after 8 weeks of therapy [6]. One patient was not evaluable due to an intracerebral hemorrhage during the first week of treatment; she had been refractory to platelet transfusions at presentation to our institution.

Of the 8 evaluable patients, none had a CR, 2 had a PR, 5 had a MR, and I had no response. Thus, 7 of 8 (88%) showed some degree of response. Of the 3 severely anemic patients, two had an improvement within 8 weeks. Of the 3 patients with platelets < 100,000/mm^3 (40,000/mm^3, 83,000/mm^3, 53,000/mm^3), all had improvement within 2 to 6 weeks (2 within 4 weeks). All 8 patients had been neutropenic; 6 had resolution at a period of 5 to 9 weeks (median 7 weeks). The HCI had decreased in 7 of the 8 patients by 8 weeks reflecting the decreased amount of hairy cells in the bone marrow after interferon treatment.

Toxicity was relatively mild. All 8 patients had fever associated with the first several injections, but rarely higher than 38.5°C. Seven patients complained of fatigue, 5 of myalgias, and 5 of drymouth. Four patients had an influenza-like syndrome that included headache, chills, low back pain, and nausea. Three patients had asymptomatic chemical hepatitis, 2 complained of abnormal taste, 2 of paresthesia, and 1 of alopecia. Of the 7 remaining patients, transient myelo-suppression was noted in 5 with a decrease in granulocyte count of a mean of 200/mm^3 around 1–2 weeks after treatment initiation and lasting for 2 weeks. Of 5 patients not receiving platelet transfusions, there was a decrease in the platelet count for a mean of 80,000/mm^3 around 1–2 weeks after treatment initiation and lasting approximately 4 weeks. Of 5 patients not receiving RBC transfusions, 3 had a decrease in their hemoglobin of a mean of 1.3 g/dl around 7 weeks after treatment initiation and lasting approximately 7 weeks.

Discussion and comparative trials

The preliminary results from the University of Chicago are very encouraging [6]. This is the first report of significant responses in HCL with recombinant alpha-2 interferon. The original report by Quesada et al [5] utilized partially purified interferon alpha. They utilized it as it had been shown to induce regression in patients with B cell neoplasms and various solid tumors with slow proliferative capacity. It has previously been shown by Braylan et al. that less than 1/2 of 1% of the hairy cells were labelled with tritiated thymidine [7]. This confirmed a very slow proliferative capacity.

A follow-up study by Quesada et al. [8] reported a total of 16 patients who received 3 million units daily by intramuscular injection. Three patients achieved a CR, 9 a PR, and 3 patients a MR. Most striking was that the bone marrow infiltrate disappeared or was reduced greater than 50% in all responsive patients and the bone marrow granulocytes increased from a median pretreatment of 10% (0–25%) to a median of 48% (29–66%) after treatment.

Besides the responses in 7 of the 8 patients from the University of Chicago, Jacobs and Golde have documented the same type of results in their study at UCLA using recombinant alpha-2 interferon [9]. They have 8 patients who finished 8 weeks of therapy; one of these patients died of intracerebral hemorrhage after one week of therapy. Six of their 8 patients had a platelet count < 100,000/mm³; after 8 weeks, 7 of 8 had a platelet count > 100,000/mm³. They also saw a dramatic increase in the percentage of granulocytes (5 of 8 had > 50% granulocytes after 8 weeks).

It appears that both partially purified alpha interferon and recombinant alpha-2 interferon have similar beneficial therapeutic effects in patients with progressive hairy cell leukemia. Even patients who have progressive disease post-splenectomy and post-chlorambucil seem to benefit significantly from interferon. Patients who have not undergone splenectomy also have shown a response, however there is still not enough evidence to suggest that treatment with interferon should replace the role of splenectomy. One has to remember that approximately two-thirds of patients will not need further treatment for long periods or at all after splenectomy. Since we do not yet know how interferon works in this disease, or how long we must continue interferon to maintain its effect, or how long we can maintain it even if its effect is beneficial, it is not yet time to advance this treatment beyond patients with progressieve disease unless a careful, controlled clinical study is being undertaken. It appears, however, that interferon should be the initial therapy choice for patients with progressive hairy cell leukemia rather than chlorambucil. Although chlorambucil has been shown to improve the anemia and thrombocytopenia at 3 to 6 months after treatment initiation by decreasing the HCI, it rarely improves the granulocytopenia, and infectious complications persist. The responses with IFN are rapid, resulting in a dramatic improvement in the absolute granulocyte count within approximately 2 months. It is possible that initial treatment with IFN followed after 3 months by the addition of chlorambucil could result in a better complete remission rate than either alone; this combination remains to be tested.

References

1. Burke JS: The value of the bone-marrow biopsy in the diagnosis of hairy cell leukemia. Am J Clin Pathol 70:876-884, 1978.
2. Mintz V, Golomb HM: Splenectomy as initial therapy in twenty-six patients with leukemic reticuloendotheliosis (hairy cell leukemia). Cancer Res 39:2366-2370, 1979.
3. Golomb HM, Vardiman JW: Response to splenectomy in 65 patients with hairy cell leukemia. An evaluation of spleen weight and bone marrow involvement. Blood 61:349-352, 1983.
4. Golomb HM: Progress report on chlorambucil therapy in post-splenectomy patients with progressive hairy cell leukemia. Blood 57:464-467, 1981.

5. Quesada JR, Reuben J, Manning JT *et al.:* Induction of remission in hairy cell leukemia with alpha interferon. N Eng J Med 310:15-18, 1984.

6. Ratain M, Jacobs R, Golomb HM: Treatment of hairy cell leukemia with recombinant alpha-2 interferon. Submitted.

7. Braylan R, Fowlkes BJ, Jaffee ES *et al.:* Structural and functional properties of the 'hairy' cells of leukemic reticuloendotheliosis. Cancer 41:201-209, 1978.

8. Quesada JR, Hirsh EM, Gutterman JV: Treatment of hairy cell leukemia with alpha interferon. Proc Am Soc Oncol II:207, 1984.

9. Jacobs A, Golde DW: Unpublished.

10. Clinical Trials in Non-Hematologic Malignancies

R.J. SPIEGEL

Abstract

In addition to trials conducted with hematologic malignancies, as presented elsewhere in these proceedings, a variety of Phase II trials have been conducted in other sarcomas and carcinomas which may provide interesting leads regarding biological mechanisms of interferon activity as well as clinical areas for further study. Phase II studies with INTRON as well as other interferon products have been largely negative in most adult solid tumors, e.g., breast, colon and lung. Most of these have been conducted in patients with advanced disease and may reflect inactivity against large bulky tumors rather than particular tumor types. More promising leads have been suggested in Kaposi's sarcoma, renal cell carcinoma, and melanoma. Furthermore, local-regional therapy in the case of superficial bladder tumors (intravescicular Rx) or ovarian carcinoma (intraperitoneal Rx) may provide other leads.

AIDS-related Kaposi's sarcoma was identified early as a potentially important area for biological intervention. Numerous studies have now confirmed both INTRON and other natural and recombinant interferon products to have high activity in this disease although none have consistently demonstrated improvement of the underlying immunological disorder. Nevertheless overall response rates in the other of 40–50% have been reported by a number of investigators and the response rate is considerably higher in patients with early stage disease. Moreover, these responses seem to be of long duration, in contrast to results obtained with chemotherapy. Renall cell CA is also a tumor in which numerous studies have confirmed a consistent although low response rate in the range of 15%. Similar results have been reported in metastatic malignant melanoma. In both of these settings, patients with minimal tumor burden appear to have the greatest potential for obtaining responses. These are important leads and hopefully further adjustments in dose and schedule or in combination with other therapy will yield more significant results. Results in superficial bladder cancers have also been very encouraging. Patients with carcinoma-in-situ were the group achieving the greatest benefit. Early results with intraperitoneal interferon in the treatment of ovarian cancer have also been encouraging.

Questions remain regarding the optimal biological vs. antiproliferative dose and schedule which should be utilized with interferon. However, these early Phase II studies have already demonstrated the activity of this compound when given near its MTD. There was a suggestion in these trials that differences in both dose and schedule may considerably affect response rates. In addition careful attention must be paid to the patient population at entry to avoid skewing trials positively or negatively or for confounding potentially good results in particular subgroups. Future directions include expansion of these studies in favorable prognostic groups and pursuit of early clinical leads suggesting synergistic combinations with chemotherapy and radiation.

Most new antineoplastic agents require extensive Phase II testing before the full scope of their clinical activity can be determined. This is also the case with interferon and a growing body of medical literature is now delineating which tumor types are sensitive to interferon. Generally, where activity has been reported with natural interferons, confirmatory activity has also been found with recombinant alpha-2 interferon (INTRON). These have included not only hematologic malignancies as presented elsewhere in these proceedings (e.g., low grade lymphomas, multiple myeloma, and hairy cell leukemia) but also in a variety of other sarcomas and carcinomas. These studies provide interesting leads regarding not only clinical areas for future trials but also indications of the potential biological mechanisms of interferon's activity. It remains premature to reach definitive conclusions about disease-specific activity at this point in interferon's clinical testing. In a number of malignancies it now appears that there is considerable schedule-dependence and dose-dependence which suggest that extensive testing in a variety of doses and schedules might be necessary before interferon's activity against any particular tumor type can be firmly established [1]. Additionally, it is apparent that in a variety of tumors, as described below and as presented in the myeloma studies [2], particular subgroups of patients need to be carefully evaluated to avoid prematurely discounting interferon's potential activity. Despite these caveats, it appears that in preliminary clinical trials INTRON as well as other interferon products have been largely inactive in most adult solid tumors, e.g., breast, colon, and lung cancer. Most of these studies have been conducted in patients with advanced disease and may reflect inactivity against large bulky tumors rather than particular tumor types. More promising leads have been suggested in Kaposi's sarcoma, renal cell carcinoma, and melanoma. Other promising leads in which preliminary data exists with alpha-2 interferon would include studies in carcinoid and brain tumors. Local-regional therapy in the case of superficial bladder tumors (intravesicular) or ovarian carcinoma (intraperitoneal treatment) may provide other leads [3].

The acquired immune deficiency syndrome (AIDS) was identified early as a potentially important area for immunologic intervention. Patients with this condition and the underlying malignancy of Kaposi's sarcoma have been studied extensively and numerous studies have now confirmed both INTRON and other natural and recombinant interferon products' high activity in this disease. These studies have not consistently demonstrated improvement of the underlying immunological disorder, however overall response rates in the order of 40–50% have been reported and the response rate is considerably higher in patients with early stage disease. Table 1 shows that the response rate with interferon can be dramatically different if it is administered to patients with early stage disease (89%) vs. patients in the late stages of disease (17%). Moreover the responses seen in these patients seem to be of long duration in contrast to the results obtained with chemotherapy.

Studies in renal cell carcinoma have confirmed a consistent although low response rate in the range of 10–20%. Similar results have been reported in metastic malignant melanoma. In these settings patients with minimal tumor burden appear to have the greatest potential for obtaining responses. Table 2 shows response rates in metastatic malignant melanoma trials based on whether the patient's largest measured tumor at baseline was greater than 1.5 cm. Patients with smaller tumor burdens at the initiation of treatment stand a far greater chance of obtaining a partial or complete response ($P < .005$). This form of analysis might be useful in explaining why various studies have reported discrepant results and demonstrates that studies can be strongly biased for or against interferon based on the types of patients enrolled into studies. Since metastatic melanoma and hypernephroma are diseases in which no conventional chemotherapy has high response rates, these results with interferon are important leads and hopefully adjustments in dose and schedule or in combination with other therapy may yield higher response rates. The analysis of the effects of baseline tumor burden may also serve as a rationale for conducting future studies, testing the role of interferon as adjuvant therapy even though the response rates against advanced disease might be considered of borderline activity.

Another promising clinical area involves the use of intravesicular interferon in

Table 1. Response rate in Kaposi's sarcoma patients

	Evaluable	CR	PR	NC	PD	Overall response rate
Total group	38	6	14	2	16	53%
Stage I & II	9	2	6	0	1	89%
Stage III & IV	29	4	8	2	15	41%

Table 2. Phase II INTRON trials in metastatic melanoma: Responses by maximum tumor size

	N	CR/PR
< 1.5 cm	26	8 (31%)
≥ 1.5 cm	40	3 (8%)

patients with superficial bladder cancers [3]. Patients with carcinoma *in situ* appear to be the group receiving the greater benefit with a high rate of complete resolution as confirmed by biopsy. Patients with papillary tumors had a lower response rate; however, these patients had tumors left in place and most trials with other intravesicular agents have been done in a setting of adjuvant treatment following surgical resection.

Obviously, with intravesicular administration high local concentrations of interferon can be obtained while systemic toxicity is avoided. No local toxicity was seen in these early trials. Further confirmatory studies are ongoing in this area.

Another result that has emerged in trials with melanoma involves the effects of schedule. When given as a daily dose ×5 every three weeks, low response rates were obtained in the treatment of metastatic malignant melanoma. However, when the same group of investigators switched to a dosing schedule which involved 3×/wk continuous dosing a consistent response rate in the range of 17–25% was obtained [4]. *In vitro* studies have predicted that continuous exposure may be necessary to obtain optimal results with interferon, and these studies with melanoma appear to confirm this (Table 3).

A strict dose–response relationship has not been confirmed in any clinical studies to date with INTRON. However, early results in Kaposi's sarcoma suggest that some threshold dose might be critical. Table 4 demonstrates the difference in response rates between a very low-dose and very high-dose administration schedule. The low-dose regimen resulted in patients obtaining fewer responses. In addition, responses required longer duration of treatment to occur. Finally, three out of four patients who switched from low-dose interferon to high-dose became responders on the high-dose. This suggests that some doses might be too low to produce responses; however, they do not establish a minimal dose which is necessary. Other studies suggest that in some malignancies quite low doses ($1-2 \times 10^6$ IU/m^2) may be adequate to produce anti-tumor effects [5].

Phase II studies have begun to clarify the true clinical role of alpha-2 interferon in a variety of malignancies. Questions remain regarding the optimal biological versus antiproliferative dose as well as the schedule which should be utilized with interferon. However, these early Phase II studies have already demonstrated the activity of INTRON when given near its maximum tolerated dose. These trials also suggest that differences in both dose and schedule may considerably affect response rates. In addition, careful attention must be paid to the patient popula-

Table 3. Phase II INTRON trials in metastatic melanoma; Responses* in 3 schedules

	N	CR	PR	NC	PD	Response rate
3–30 mu/m² IV daily	13	2	0	2	9	15.4%
30 mu/m² IV qd × 5/3 wks	30	0	1	4	25	3.3%
10 mu/m² sq tiw	64	3	8	6	47	17.2%

* Response required two confirmatory measurements 4 weeks apart.

Table 4. Phase II INTRON trials in Kaposi's sarcoma: High vs. low dose

	Evaluable patients	Response				Percent response
		CR	PR	NC	PD	
High dose						
50 million IU/m^2	29	4	10	2	13	48.3%
Low dose						
1 million IU/m^2	9	1	2	0	2	33.3%
Low initial dose						
High maintenance	4	1	2	0	1	75.0%
Overall dose	38	6	14	2	16	52.6%

tion at entry to avoid skewing trials positively or negatively, or confounding potentially good results in particular subgroups. Future directions for interferon clinical trials include expansion of these studies in favorable prognostic groups, pursuing preclinical leads suggesting synergistic combinations of different interferons (e.g. alpha & gamma) or combining alpha interferon with chemotherapeutic agents or radiation therapy.

References

1. Sonnenfeld G: Contradictory results in interferon research. Surv Immunol Res 3:198-201, 1984.
2. Costanzi, *et al.* Lugano Symposium.
3. Torti FM, Shortliffe LD, Williams RD, Spaulding JT, Hannigan JF Jr, Palmer J, Myers FJ, Higgins M, Freiha FS: Superficial bladder cancer responsive to alpha-2 interferon administered intravesically.
4. Robinson WA, Kirkwood JM, Harvey H, Mughal T, McCune C, Muggia F, Hawkins M, Muscato M, Pouillart P, Ernstoff M, Sorell M, Spiegel R: Effective use of recombinant human alpha-2 interferon in metastic malignant melanoma.
5. Golomb, *et al.* Lugano Symposium.

11. Discussion: Clinical Panel

J.F. SMYTH and PARTICIPANTS

Dr. Berneman, Antwerp: I have a question for Dr. Spiegel. Is there any cardiac toxicity of interferon whatsoever and would you consider giving interferon to a person with cardiac disease? I ask you this question because we witnessed a case where a patient with known ischemic heart disease and complete left bundle branch block on EKG received interferon. Two weeks after starting treatment, he suddenly died at home; he did not receive his interferon that day.

Dr. Spiegel: This is obviously a very important question. As you and some members of the audience may know, there were early reports from French studies of presumed cardiac toxicity. They were not using recombinant interferon, but other interferons. These reports have not been published and we have not seen exactly to what the data refers, however we have looked very extensively to make sure that we are not, in fact, missing an important toxicity. I would make two comments; one is that our clinical protocols at present exclude patients who have known cardiac abnormalities and who definitely require medication. Our major concern is that we have a 90 percent plus incidence of fevers, in some cases very high fevers, and I think a considerable number of patients get sinus tachycardia simply because we have elevated their body temperature. We have not had any evidence that interferon, in any other way, is a direct arrhythogenic agent. The only other problem we have seen were episodes of hypotension, which in 8 out of 9 cases to date responded very promptly to fluid replacement. We feel these patients were initially dehydrated. I would invite my other collaborators here who have had first-hand experience, to mention anything else they have seen. We do not presently believe that interferon alpha-2 is cardiotoxic.

Dr. Smyth: Does anyone else on the panel want to comment on cardiotoxicity?

Dr. Wagstaff: In Manchester we had two patients with problems; one patient had a history of angina and he described quite clearly that, on the day that he had his interferon, his angina was worse. In fact he subsequently had a myocardial infarction. The other patient who had previously had cardiac arrhythmias was given only three injections of interferon. She was admitted and died from an intractable arrhythmia.

Dr. Smyth: Was that related to hyperthermia?

Dr. Wagstaff: Well, both of those patients were receiving the 2 million units of interferon, so the fevers they had were minor.

Dr. Misset, Villevif, France: We were not involved in the study where cardiac toxicities were observed. However, we have some more information. It appears that those patients who had cardiac toxicity in Paris, were given interferon shortly after adriamycin courses. Dr. Shallshanee has developed a mouse model in which he observed cardiac toxicity if interferon was given to mice shortly after anthracyclines. After what we have heard this afternoon, I think we had better give interferon before anthracyclines. Now I have a question for Dr. Golomb: I would like to challenge part of your statement that early patients should not be treated with interferon when they have hairy-cell leukemia. Do you think this is a temporary statement, or is it definitive? I do not think we have had any instances in malignant disease where you do not get better results when treating early patients rather than late patients.

Dr. Golomb: The challenge is a worthy one because while I would make that statement now, I would not say that it is absolute. I say that because we do not know how long we can treat patients with interferon. What happens if they become resistant or if they are not able to tolerate interferon? You have seen one of the speakers show that patients are developing some skin reactions to interferon. We have observed that now in two patients after 6 or 7 months. It does not seem to be serious, but there could be a problem. Therefore, not knowing how long a patient should be treated with interferon, or what the long-term effects are, I feel that we should not begin to treat patients early on with it until we know a little more about how patients do later. I think the question that has to be asked is, can we treat patients prior to splenectomy with interferon and what happens? We have hae one patient recently who came in with a platelet count of 40,000, a one centimeter palpable spleen below the costal margin and he refused splenectomy. We started him immediately on interferon. After about 8 weeks his platelet count was a little over 100,000. It is not the dramatic response that we saw in other patients who were post-splenectomy, but we do have one patient treated early. Therefore, I think that in the future in a controlled setting, we should look at earlier patients. However, I do not want to advocate for the general population of new hairy cell patients, who have not yet undergone splenectomy, treatment with interferon at this time.

Dr. Hagberg, Uppsala, Sweden: We have treated 11 patients with hairy cell leukemia and have hae the same good results that you have described. One of our problems is that within the first two or three weeks we have many infections. Four or five patients have had severe infections at the beginning of the treatment. My question is, have you had the same experience?

Dr. Golomb: No, we have not seen the early infections. One of the requirements of entry has been no active infection and not on antibiotics. Therefore, patients have not been infected when they started. We have noted fever that has persisted in only one patient out of the first 21. He had 5 days of fever in Colorado, we then had him flown to Chicago, where on arrival he was afebrile without a source and looked fine. There has been a real absence of fever or infectious complications in patients who have started interferon, and that has surprised me, but this is consistent with the Quesada data at this time. Maybe Dr. Hofmann would like to comment?

Dr. Hofmann: I have the same findings as Dr. Golomb. In the study of the Swiss patients no one has any infectious complications, although one had severe and repeated infections before treatment was started. Of the other European cases, there were no infections.

Dr. Hagberg: In one of your slides there was at first a decrease in the neutrophils before the increase occurred.

Dr. Hofmann: I mentioned that the patient had only one value above one thousand and that was the day we started treatment. Previous to that measurement, counts were below 500.

Dr. Ruco, Rome: I have a question for the hairy cell leukemia presenters. I want to know if interferon has any definite effect on hairy cells *in vitro*. Have they noticed any change, prior to or after the interferon treatment, in the hairy cells of the patient?

Dr. Golomb: The *in vitro* studies that we have done have only been over the last three months. To perform *in vitro* studies you need patients with a high peripheral count and as I had shown you earlier we had only five. We examined two spleens. We only had evidence in one patient that there was any *in vitro* killing at seven days and it happened to be the first patient of the series. The subsequent three patients studied have shown no differences between the control and the *in vitro* interferon treatment. On the other hand, we have had a long interest in the ultrastructural aspects of the hairy cell, and have looked at the nature of cytoplasmic organelles within the hairy cells. We have found the induction of tubular reticular structures (TRS'), which have been described before in patients treated with interferon in immune disorders. We have found the induction of these complexes within the hairy cells, because we can find them in cells that have ribosomal lamellar complexes. We do not find the induction of these in all cases at this point, which suggests to us that there could be a correlation between the induction of these and subsequent response. There are a number of phenomena that are occurring about which we have some clues, but we do not have enough cases to answer our questions conclusively.

Dr. Ruco: Did you look at the surface antigens of the cell?

Dr. Golomb: Initially we looked at the surface immunoglobulins, but not subsequently. One of the problems later in treatment is that there are very few cells to look at by one month, as I mentioned earlier, because of the drop in the leukemic cell count.

Dr. Hofmann: In Zurich, about 4 years ago, we devised a clonogenic assay to clone hairy cells. They grew very well following stimulation with PHALCM. In some of them we have looked at the effect of interferon *in vitro* and found some very dramatic inhibition of hairy cell leukemia growth. So, there is a hint that interferon may be cytotoxic to hairy cells, but I do not know anything else about the mechanism of action.

Dr. Schwartzmeier, Vienna: If you would permit, I would like to show two slides on studies we were just performing with hairy cell leukemia. We are currently studying the effects of various chemotherapeutic agents on the *in vitro* incorporation of tritiated uridine and thymidine, in order to assess the sensitivity or the inhibitory effect of these agents. What we are currently looking at is the *in vitro* sensitivity, as measured by the inhibition of incorporation of uridine and thymidine by various agents. We also looked at interferon. With this short-term assay (incubation is only for three hours with interferon), we did not find any appreciable inhibition of nucleoside precursor incorporation. However, in the next slide I would like to show you the *in vivo* results with interferon treatment with one of these patients. As with the other investigators we had the same type of good response: hairy cells are reduced, hemoglobin, red blood cells and platelets are increased. We have had the same good *in vivo* experience in Vienna.

Dr. Salem, Lebanon: Dr. Spiegel, would you like to comment on the effects of interferon in renal cell carcinoma?

Dr. Spiegel: That is certainly one of the diseases in which there has been great interest since interferon became available for widespread clinical testing. In fact, there have been quite discrepant results and it has been difficult for us to determine whether the differences between reports, including our own, reflect differences in interferon preparations, in the dose and schedule utilized or in the type of patients. Overall we feel that we have a very large experience. Some of the early reports were small studies of 20–30 patients using either other recombinant interferon products or natural interferon and my own reading of the literature shows that the general range of objective response is about 15–25% of patients. In our own experience in the Schering trials, as has been reported in a number of meetings by this time, our overall response rates are only in the range of 10%. However, I would note that the patients in our own trials were recruited with very few exclusions. We treated patients with very advanced disease, they were allowed to have extensive prior chemotherapy and to have metastases at any site. Some of the more positive results have come from studies where patients with known metastases were excluded, patients had no prior therapy or only one prior therapy, and favorable performance status. Therefore, I think ours is a real response rate. Dr. Leavitt, who has done some of the renal studies with us, might wish to comment further. There is some real activity, I think, with interferon by itself. It is a rather low level of activity, and is one of those areas that might be particularly interesting to use interferon in combination with other drugs, given that no drugs have particularly high response rates in renal cell carcinoma.

Dr. Smyth: I think that with one of the points that came up earlier in the afternoon is to decide what to call interferon; is this a drug? If you call it a "biological response modifier", that does not really mean anything other than a descriptive term for a compound that is being tested in man. Conventionally, we are all attuned to assessing response very early on. Therefore, we tend to assess a drug or compound as not being effective if the response is not observed early on.

This is the case with alpha-2 and with some of the other experimental cytotoxic compounds. However, if you have a disease that is not progressing so rapidly, you may see that responses (for example in diseases such as melanoma and renal cell cancer) at times quite divorced from the usual times at which drugs are assessed.

Dr. Spiegel: Let me add, that when I talk about response rates, I am used to conventionally being very strict and only defining responses as pure complete responses, or partial responses as 50% decreases in tumor size. One of the first reports on renal cell that was very exciting, was Dr. Guttermann's, where he also included patients with stable disease. We have tried not to do that. However at the recent ASCO meetings, Dr. Kempf, an investigator at the University of Southern California, showed that 50% of the patients on our Schering trial with renal cell carcinoma had stable disease after treatment, when all had progressive disease at the time they started therapy. I have tried not to mix various types of responses together. I believe Dr. Leavitt would like to comment further.

Dr. Leavitt: Those are really the only comments that I would want to make: We also did not count patients who had mixed responses in which some tumors got smaller and some tumors got larger. I think that is scientifically correct to do, but it does show in those patients there is some biological effect that may be of importance with smaller bulk disease.

Dr. Zwitter, Lubijana: I have a question for Dr. Kisner. You know that some spontaneous remissions of untreated Hodgkin's disease after measles have been reported. Would you agree that this may be due to endogenous interferon secretion and do you see any potential use of that in therapy?

Dr. Kisner: It would be impossible to say that this is not the case. However, it is fair to point out that most patients do not have measurable levels of circulating interferon and nothing near the therapeutic levels achieved in these studies. I certainly can not say for sure that we did not have spontaneous remissions in the Hodgkin's disease trial. I suspect we did not. In addition to the three partial responses out of 13 evaluable patients, we saw biological activity in the form of mixed responses in four additional patients. Considering the degree of prior therapy, this was surprising to us and convinces us that the material has activity in Hodgkin's disease requiring further study.

Dr. Zwitter: I think for measles, the measles vaccine was suggested as a possible addition to conventional therapy.

Dr. Kisner: As an interferon inducer?

Dr. Zwitter: Yes.

Dr. Kisner: I think there is no question that viral infections and vaccines can induce interferon as well as a variety of other known interferon inducers.

Dr. Heinz, Vienna: I am particularly interested in Dr. Leavitt's patient who died early because of gastrointestinal bleeding. In my very limited experience with interferon, I treated a patient with Burkitt's lymphoma. I was confronted with inexplicable, severe gastrointestinal bleeding. The patient was not thrombocytopenic, I would like to ask you for an explanation of your patient's bleeding.

Dr. Leavitt: In the large number of patients that I have treated at several doses, with different kinds of cancer, that was the only patient I have seen that had severe gastrointestinal bleeding. In retrospect, she had symptoms of indigestion that predated the beginning of the interferon trial. My suspicion is that she had a peptic ulcer or gastritis before we treated her. I am not sure that interferon was responsible. On the other hand, another patient who had immunoblastic sarcoma, and who had stable disease through 4 or 5 cycles of treatment, did develop some hematochezia and oral ulceration. I am certain that this was a result of mucositis from interferon treatment and we listed that as toxicity.

Dr. Spiegel: I might add that I only listed on my summary toxicity slides toxicities that appeared with a $> 5\%$ incidence, or very severe toxicities. We examined carefully in Phase I trials the coagulation profiles of prothrombin and partial thromboplastin times. We saw no consistant coagulopathies during interferon treatment, either acutely or chronically.

Unidentified speaker: I have a question concerning combined interferon and chemotherapy. What is the rationale for giving interferon one hour before doxorubicin and then giving a two-hour infusion of doxorubicin? Is this based on some data, or just an idea. What is the reason for it?

Dr. Spiegel: Dr. Welander's study was designed to give a maximal level of interferon at the time the adriamycin was given. He gives an interferon IV bolus and then simultaneously gives a SC injection in order to obtain a high level of interferon rapidly. Two hours later he gives doxorubicin. As far as mechanisms of action, nothing is known. There is the potential that interferon may affect the surface membrane, and it may effect the influx or the egress of a cytotoxic drug. It may produce some type of cycling effects. We know that it alters the way tumor cells and normal cells go through the cell cycle. There are a number of possible explanations, but we do not know the exact mechanism of synergy.

Dr. Kisner: I have a question for Dr. Spiegel: You showed the data on melanoma regarding the response rates and tumor nodule size, and mentioned that this might be a rationale for use in minimal residual disease or in a surgical adjuvant setting. I think that would be true for any chemotherapy agent in any tumor type as well. Few oncologists would be willing to put into the surgical adjuvant setting a drug, for example, that had a 10% or a 5% response rate in advanced disease. I wonder if you could comment on that.

Dr. Spiegel: We all know that with most chemotherapy, we expect patients with minimal disease to do better than patients with bulky disease. In the case of melanoma, perhaps I did not give enough background. There is clear evidence from *in vitro* models that various melanoma cell lines show sensitivity to interferon. In human tumor stem cell assays, melanoma cells have also shown sensitivity to interferon. We were encouraged, from our Phase I studies where some responses occurred, as well as other reports of clinical activity, to continue with Phase II melanoma trials. When we did the studies in the conventional population of patients with advance disease, we found activity, but at a lower level. Based on our impression, the data we had and the fact that some of the patients did achieve complete responses, we expected to see more activity in the adjuvant setting than would be expected from the overall response. I did not have a chance to present this, but for example, in ovarian cancer, it is acknowledged that patients with minimal tumor bulk, or positive cytologies only, at a second look are more likely to respond than patients with bulky abdominal disease. We have had similar results in ovarian cancer and melanoma. Before we dismiss some early trials that have only been done in heavily pretreated patients with very bulky disease, we must consider that there may be greater activity in the adjuvant setting.

Dr. Bianco, Naples: Dr. Spiegel, I was wondering whether you have or if you know of any data dealing with bladder carcinoma and papilloma?

Dr. Spiegel: Yes, there was a report at the ASCO meetings in early May presented by Dr. Frank Torti, summarizing his Phase I/II study treating superficial bladder cancers with intravesicular interferon. In that study the treated patients with papillary tumors and with carcinoma *in situ.* Papillary tumors are known to respond to a variety of intravesicular chemotherapeutic agents, but the carcinoma *in situ* is relatively resistant. He reported that approximately 7 out of 10 evaluable patients had disappearance of the carcinoma *in situ,* confirmed by biopsy. In the papillary tumors, he was treating patients who did not have resected tumors. These patients had papillary tumors left in place. He observed high activity rates in that setting. Intravesicular treatment of superficial bladder cancer appears to be an exciting area to pursue.

Dr. Bungeles, Athens: In hairy cell leukemia, after splenectomy, we may restore the blood count to normal, although the disease still exists in the bone marrow. My question for Dr. Golomb is: How sure are we that the mode of action of interferon is related to the hairy cells themselves, or may it act through a different pathway?

Dr. Golomb: After the splenectomy, there are hairy cells left in the marrow and as I pointed out, two-thirds of the patients never need treatment, although some will need treatment within three months after the splenectomy. We have recently seen some patients 14–16 years after their splenectomy who now have deteriorating blood counts. How do we know what the mechanism of the interferon is? I am not sure whether it has one or two mechanisms of action. It may act directly on the hairy cells, or it may act on other cells such as natural killer cells or it could be a combination of direct and indirect effects. I think it must be both because there is clearly a dramatic decrease in the number of hairy cells in the peripheral blood, and at the same time there is stimulation of other elements in the bone marrow. We have also seen an increase in monocytes. How that affects other cell functions, we do not know. However, I think that there are several activities occurring and clearly the patients benefit. It is possible that over the next one or two years we will found out what the reasons for this are.

Dr. Honegger, Zurich: Would the panelists comment on the neurotoxicity that obviously occurs during interferon treatment? The group that treated myeloma reported mainly a central nervous system problem. On the other hand, in patients with myeloma, do you see peripheral effects, such as paresthesias or similar problems and what is known about it?

Dr. Costanzi: In a large group of patients with myeloma that we have treated, we have seen confusion in only about 7% of the patients. We have seen no peripheral neuropathy whatsoever in any of the patients, for example parethesia or footdrop or similar complaints. It has been mainly confusion. In a few of the patients the confusion was of a severity such that they wanted to stop the therapy, but by reducing the dose the confusion cleared. We have seen no peripheral neuropathy.

Dr. Honegger: Was this dependent on the way you used the interferon?

Dr. Costanzi: No, it appeared to be related to dose. The patients who were confused were given the higher doses. We reduced the dose. If the confusion did not clear, we stopped the interferon until the confusion cleared, then we gradually reintroduced the dose. It does appear to be dose related. I might add that in our hypernephroma study, we noticed that patients became confused more frequently when they had brain metastases. I think this has been the experience of other investigators, to the point that one of our eligibility criteria is that the patient should not have brain metastases because the central nervous system toxicity is increased 10-fold over patients who do not have central nervous system metastases.

Dr. Leavitt: I think that we can predict which patients would be at high risk for confusion. They would be the elderly and those with decreased performance status, patients with brain tumors, especially if they have had previous radiotherapy, and patients with other preexisting neurological disease, especially brain disease, chronic brain syndrome from alcoholism. The confusion resolves rather slowly over a long period of time, two to three weeks. I will add that in another Phase One trial with a different recombinant interferon, I have seen true myalgia parasthetica, a lateral femoral cutaneous nerve neuropathy, that improved over two to three months. It is, I think, a rare but real toxicity of interferon. There are occasional patients who complain of numbness and tingling, which usually goes away with therapy, but I think that this may be a real toxicity of interferon.

12. Conclusion

J.F. SMYTH

We have had a very interesting afternoon. In planning the program we purposely tried to include as much as we could and inevitably we have had to go rapidly over an enormous amount of data. I hope that you have not found it too indigestible! I want to try, very briefly, to summarize just what I felt were the highlights and the areas of particular controversy.

It is clear that from the technical point of view, we are working with an extremely pure compound. This is probably very important if we adhere to the term "biological response modifier". That is certainly very far from the case in terms of other agents when these were called immunotherapeutic agents. It is also unusual in terms of cytotoxic drugs and, I think, very encouraging.

Dr. Trotta dealt with the pre-clinical data and experimental models. There is always a challenge in terms of translating the benefit and results in experimental models into clinical activity. I think the xenograft studies are clearly of interest, but there are particular problems in interpreting the data of an agent which will potentially alter immune responses in a model which depends on having an immune deficit, such as the nude mouse model. There are other difficulties, and we have heard a great deal about different ways of administering alpha-2 interferon by different ways of dosing and of scheduling. I think that it is hard to draw firm conclusions about these two parameters. I noticed that even in the nude mouse studies, some involved giving intralesional interferon. Some of the studies, such as Balkwill's from the ICRF in London, treat the mouse subcutaneously. There is no doubt that there is a significant increase in NK cell activity. I think this is an extremely important observation, indicating that alpha-2 interferon clearly is intrinsically cytotoxic. The *in vitro* studies reassure us of that. We have heard of the interesting and important work on interferon receptor characterization, with the attractive caveat that it might be possible to predict patients, particularly those who are not likely to respond. We are dealing with a compound which is definitely, in some dose schedules, toxic. If response is related to the presence of a demonstrable receptor, then by analogy with estrogen receptor data in breast in cancer management, we could select our patients for these types of studies.

Dr. Welander covered perhaps one of the most interesting areas for the future, and that is the combined use of alpha-2 interferon with conventional cytotoxic agents. The data he presented, particularly on ovarian carcinoma, were especially important. Four of 16 patients who had failed or progressed on therapy with cyclophosphamide/adriamycin/cis-platinum responded following a short exposure to interferon. Then there was a rather unusual way of administering doxorubicin over a two hour infusion. He discussed the difficulties and practicalities of not being able to extend that further but I am sure this type of approach is something that other people are going to pursue. Dr. Welander and others have referred to the studies of *in vitro* synergy that are ongoing in ovarian and breast cancer cell lines using interferon and cytotoxic drugs in the nude mouse model. I would add that in our own institution we have some interesting preliminary data on potentiation of cytotoxic drugs active against non small cell lung cancer with interferon in xenograft systems.

Dr. Spiegel, in his first presentation, gave us an excellent résumé of one of the most important aspects that we have discussed this afternoon, and that is the difficulty of designing Phase I and II studies for a biological response modifier. I think most of you would agree that the model that has been used for these studies is in fact a conventional model for assessing a new cytotoxic drug. We make a great many assumptions about cytotoxic drugs, but very often the concept of dose-response effect is seen in pre-clinical data and therefore gets explored in Phase I studies. It is by no means clear to me that there is a dose response effect of alpha-2 interferon in man and therefore I think, as Dr. Spiegel pointed out, we have to be appropriately critical of our own study designs in the Phase I and II settings. He observed the obvious difficulty of choosing appropriate patients and the difficulties of working with patients who have been heavily pre-treated, when one might expect additional toxicities. Dr. Spiegel thought that the pre-clinical data was of little relevance as regards to biological response modifiers, but I do not feel quite as strongly as that. I think that some of the pre-clinical data is helpful but I quite agree that there is a large gap to be bridged. The most important point relates to the scheduling of the drug rather than to the absolute dose, where if you are hoping to achieve a sustained augmentation of the biological effect, almost certainly the chronicity of the therapy is just as important as the dose that is given. The pharmacokinetic studies that he refered to tend to support that point.

Dr. Wagstaff gave the first of the talks on lymphoma, in which a variety of different regimes have been used for treating high grade and low grade lymphoma. Three partial responses out of 10 patients with high grade lymphoma and a 38% overall response in low grade lymphoma were reported, although responses tended to be of rather short duration. Again, the obvious point, particularly with the low grade lymphomas, is that the design of therapy is critically important. We are looking for therapeutic design which allows for chronic exposure rather than a tendency to use high dose short-term therapy for the most aggressive lymphomas.

In the studies that Dr. Leavitt presented from five centers in the U.S., there were short, but definite responses in low grade lymphomas. Three partial responses were seen in 13 patients form Maryland and five partial responses and one complete response were seen in 17 patients from the other centers. The high grade lymphoma regime presented from other U.S. centers was much more toxic and used a much higher dose of interferon; three partial responses were seen in 29 patients with only one complete response. This was an interesting patient with T cell diffuse undifferentiated lymphoma, the response lasting for over 18 months.

Dr. Kisner reviewed data on 13 evaluable patients with Hodgkin's disease in which there were three responses, two were nodular sclerosing and one had mixed cellularity. Although these responses were of short duration (3-5 months), these were patients who had been heavily pre-treated. Dr. Kisner emphasized that, accepting there is activity in Hodgkin's disease, we should look at the treatment of refractory patients who have not been too heavily pre-treated.

Dr. Costanzi presented a very careful analysis of data from 38 patients with myeloma. The obvious problem that came to me from the analysis was the difficulty of defining a dose and a schedule. He looked at three different doses, ranging from a very low dose of three million units to one hundred million units, in three different ways. Dr. Costanzi was the only person who presented evidence suggesting that the toxicities of those three different regimes were similar. My impression from the afternoon's proceedings was that toxicity is clearly related to dose. We certainly found this in our own studies. Whether or not efficacy is related to dose I am not certain. However, my impressions with the data to date is that this is not proven. I think duration of exposure to therapy irrespective of dose appears to be more important, and obviously patient tolerance is better if the doses are low.

We have heard some fascinating data about hairy cell leukemia. It is not extraordinary in terms of biological responses that we keep developing effective therapies for very rare cancers, but we cannot solve the problem of the common cancers. Here again, except in Chicago, we are talking about a rare disease. Fortunately, Dr. Golomb shared with us his experience, which must be the most extensive experience in the world now in hairy cell leukemia. I thought the responses were extremely exciting. These results were supported by the case histories from Dr. Hofmann. By analogy with other rare cancers we have often learned the most important lessons from studying the rare cancers. I think the model of hairy cell leukemia in man presents to us some very interesting examples of how we might explore the activity of interferon in human diseases. Here we have a disease where time may be on our side. It is not necessary to treat all patients. We can select when to treat only some of the patients, and it may very well be the case in a few years time that we have learned an enormous number of lessons from the studies in hairy cell.

Dr. Spiegel summarized some of the data on the treatment of other tumors and made some important points about not being too pessimistic about negative results in cancers for which we have very little to offer, such as renal cell cancer and malignant melanoma. Of course, he emphasized the importance that in reporting data, it is only fair to adhere to conventional criteria.

However, if one is looking for clues, some of the minor responses that have been reported must be interpreted in light of the fact that they are only minor responses, but they may give us important clues in the future. Dr. Spiegel summarized the data on Kaposi's sarcoma with a 53% response rate. I think it is fair to say that Dr. Spiegel was keen on emphasizing that we now know that there are dose and schedule determinants which will help us with further studies. My own feeling is that we still have a great deal to learn with regard to this. It is clear that there is no single dose or schedule which stands out in any of the various trials and, if my arithmetic is correct, we have heard of at least 12 different ways of giving alpha-2 interferon this afternoon.

So what about the future? I believe we have two possible scenarios which immediately come to mind. The first is that we have a group of tumors in which alpha-2 interferon clearly has activity and those are predominantly the lymphomas, the hematological malignancies, hairy cell leukemia, and Kaposi's sarcoma. In these cancers I would suggest that the next important work is to try to define what is the optimal duration and dose of therapy. My own bias is towards studies which will allow us in terms of patient compliance and toxicity to pursue the chronicity of therapy. The other group of cancers are the cancers for which there has been either no response or only minor responses. These are the cancers, especially in the latter group where there have been minor responses, in which I think we will be looking for synergism with cytotoxic drugs. For some of those cancers, the work on tumor models is likely to be very helpful to us. Underlying all of this is the need to find out what alpha-2 interferon and the other interferons actually do in terms of both the potentiating effect they have on cytotoxic drugs and on killing tumor cells in their own right. Dr. Spiegel gave us an excellent résumé of all the possible mechanisms in which alpha-2 interferon might have a cytotoxic effect. Although it is becoming clear that the minimum requirement is to have a receptor on the cell's surface, what the form of gene amplification or gene product produced as a result of interferon binding with the malignant cell is yet to be understood. The more we understand about the actual mechanism of action and particularly the critical target within the cell, the more likely we are to learn how best to use what seems to me to be a most interesting and promising product.

Finally, in closing this part of the meeting, I would like to thank the organizers, particularly those from the Schering-Plough Corp. who have put in a great deal of work to organize this afternoon. I couple that with thanks to Franco Cavalli who introduced us earlier on this afternoon. Those of you who have been involved in organizing similar meetings know what an extraordinary amount of activity takes place over many months before an event, which then only takes four to five hours. So on behalf of Dr. Kisner and myself, I would like to thank the organizers at Schering-Plough very much indeed and thank all of you for your participation this afternoon.